INFLAMED

INFLAMED

discover the root cause of inflammation and personalize a step-by-step plan to create a healthy, vibrant life

BY SHELLY MALONE, MPH, RDN

Paperback ISBN: 978-0-692-70440-0

Agustin Publishing
Printed in the United States

Cover design by Melody Christian
Back cover photograph by Nicola Borland

www.inflamedbook.com
www.shellymalone.com

To Jordan, my angel.

Thank you for choosing me.

TABLE OF CONTENTS

PART FOUR: TOOLKIT

INTRODUCTION:

HOT AND BOTHERED

I had inadvertently set myself on fire.

Everything about me was hot and bothered. I was consumed by inflammation — overwhelming fatigue, painful joints and burning skin — and it was taking me down.

Once I figured out what I was in the throes of — a chronic, inflammatory (and in my case, autoimmune) condition — I realized I was hot and bothered in other ways, too. Angry at the lack of transparent, helpful information available to me. Frustrated by subtleties and nuances that aimed to confuse. Irritated by conflicting statistics and stories I read.

So I forged my own path, and found my own way to feel better. I've reclaimed good health and yet...I'm still troubled by the subject. If as a master's trained registered dietitian I didn't have the information to address my condition with diet and lifestyle, I could only imagine how difficult it must be for someone without a background in health or nutrition looking for relief from their symptoms. On my journey I learned that unless you have the time, resources and ability to forge a path less traveled — research progressive practices, and pay for services outside of conventional healthcare — you won't find the answers you need.

If you are suffering and searching — as I was — for a way to heal naturally from a chronic condition, consider that you are now holding in your hands a new, concise guide to changing your life by reducing inflammation.

This book is for those diagnosed with a chronic disease, autoimmune or otherwise. And it is for anyone without a specific diagnosis, but enduring chronic symptoms like fatigue, aches and pains, digestive or skin issues and not finding relief with conventional care.

In the following pages, you'll discover the root cause of your issues and a path to better health:

- In **Part One: Fire Hazard**, you'll learn how your genetics, digestion and the environment act as kindling for the fire of inflammation.
- In **Part Two: Ignition**, you'll discover which factors of your diet, lifestyle, environment (internal and external) and medical history are stoking the fire.
- In **Part Three: Extinguish**, you will implement a personalized, step-by-step action plan to put out the flames.

Before we get started, let me share how I got here.

THERE HAS TO BE A BETTER WAY

I remember sitting on my couch searching "rheumatoid arthritis" on the internet the day my blood work confirmed my diagnosis. The first statistic that came racing to my eye was from a Johns Hopkins study, "sixty percent of people with rheumatoid arthritis will be unable to work 10 years after disease onset." Come again? Not be able to *work?* I am glued to a chair in front of a computer screen, on a plane, or in meetings most of the day. In 10 years, I won't be able to do *that?* The tears started to flow. I was just 32 years old with a 6-week old baby girl.

Prior to this, I would have been considered an extremely healthy gal — a registered dietitian (RD) by trade, a competitive athlete, never receiving anything short of a glowing bill of health. Now I was faced with a chronic, autoimmune disease without reliable indicators to predict how quickly it would progress. I was scared and devastated, with the countdown to debilitation ticking loudly in my head. I woke every morning with my body on fire, feeling like I had a never-ending flu, and I was so tired I couldn't get out of bed. My knuckles were so swollen that I couldn't get my wedding ring on and my wrists and hands were in so much pain that I couldn't hold my daughter to breastfeed.

I indulged in a pretty elaborate pity party while the words of my demoralizing rheumatologist ("you should feel lucky you're not in a wheelchair") rang loudly in my head. But my baby girl and my off-the-charts Type-A personality quickly motivated me to find the answers I needed to beat this thing...answers other than long-term steroids and immunosuppressant medications. Their laundry lists of side effects include glaucoma, osteoporosis, weight gain and "moon face," mood swings, increased infection risk and nutrient deficiencies. Reading them almost made the rheumatoid arthritis (RA) sound pretty good. In what universe does RA + steroids = vibrant health? Was I really supposed to fill up on medication and feel like a puffer fish, or else be in debilitating pain? These were my only options??

After an underwhelming experience with conventional medicine, I explored more progressive options and in doing so, learned about the havoc food sensitivities can wreak on your system, as well as the principles of an anti-inflammatory diet. What should be concerning (for everyone) is that as a RD (now referred to as a RDN, registered dietitian nutritionist), a bachelor's degree in Nutrition *and* a master's degree in Nutrition and Public Health, this information about the critical role food plays in inflammation came as headline news to me:

- *Anti-inflammatory diet?* Never heard of it.
- *Eliminate gluten if you don't have celiac disease?* Why?
- *The function of your immune system is largely based on the effectiveness of your digestive system.* Huh?
- *Eliminate toxins that can come from non-organic foods and artificial sweeteners, additives and preservatives?* That's a load of alternative health crap.

The first obstacle after fully educating myself was *what the hell am I supposed to eat*? I used my education (and desperation) to wade through all the questions, and nutritional guidelines, and how many different words companies are allowed to use in an ingredients list so that they don't have to explicitly tell you it could cause harm.

I even started my own food company — Clean Cravings — and in the process developed a unique perspective on the allergy-free, gluten-free, natural food industry. I kept my mind and my eyes open, and I realized that the new foods I was putting into my body weren't just good for my rheumatoid arthritis, they were good for my whole being. Other chronic issues I had previously suffered from — sinus infections, migraines, depression — were also falling away.

My new clean, anti-inflammatory principles quickly expanded beyond diet and into most every other aspect of my life as I continued my research. I am not bathed in patchouli oil or healing crystals (not that I judge), but I became quite discerning with the personal care and other products within my home to lower the overall toxic load to my system. I use nutrition, acupuncture, physical therapy and/or mind-body work for any minor physical ailments to avoid medications that may be harmful to my system. I use targeted supplementation to address nutrient deficiencies I have due to my genetic variations. I still have great respect for the advances from Western medicine, and you better believe I'll be racing to the hospital if any serious, acute medical event occurs. However, I believe strongly in the body's ability to heal itself. And more than anything, I believe in finding and resolving the root cause of the issue, rather than relying solely on a quick, pharmacological fix.

Over 50 million Americans suffer from an autoimmune disease — with numbers on the rise—and 50 percent of our adults AND children are living with a chronic health condition. And yet, our current health system is doing society a huge disservice. Moving towards an anti-inflammatory lifestyle — altering the foods we eat and the products we put in, on and around our bodies, lowering stress—plays a huge role in managing not only autoimmune conditions, but almost all chronic conditions, and that fact has been largely ignored.

That's why I wrote this book. To communicate — louder than the mainstream messages and outdated conventional paradigms — the power behind progressive diet and lifestyle changes to address the root cause of the issue: inflammation. I believe there has to be a better way.

It's time to get hot and bothered about being hot and bothered.

PART ONE
FIRE HAZARD

CHAPTER 1:

INFLAMMATION EXPOSED

When your body is taken over by inflammation, it can not only be debilitating, it can raise your risk for heart disease, diabetes, obesity, some cancers, mood and cognitive disorders and is the source of autoimmune disease and many other chronic conditions.

And when almost one-half of all Americans (and 50% of our children) live with some type of chronic health condition and 38 million people across the globe die each year from preventable "lifestyle disease," it is time for us to take notice and put some energy towards addressing the root cause of the issue.

What is a Lifestyle Disease?

The term lifestyle disease refers to any chronic disease that could have been prevented by changes in one's lifestyle – diet, exercise habits, tobacco use, stress, and environmental factors. Basically, this includes any chronic disease that is not considered communicable (or contagious). Some examples include: type 2 diabetes, obesity, many cardiovascular diseases (e.g. atherosclerosis, hypertension), some liver and renal (kidney) disease, many cancers. Historically, this has been a category of disease that has not been a focus for the global health agenda. It has been referred to as "the social justice issue of our time."

INFLAMMATION DEFINED

Simply put, inflammation is the immune system's response to a stimulus that is viewed as foreign or toxic to your body (also known as an antigen). Your immune system constantly monitors for anything that appears as a foreign intruder (like an infectious bacteria or other material) that shouldn't be in the body, and is always at the ready to signal its highly-specialized troops of cells and molecules to attack and dispose of the foreign material.

Inflammation can play a positive role in our health as the primary defense mechanism against acute conditions — like when a fever fights off an infection, or blood rushes to a sprained ankle to help heal the tissue. It is an essential part of healing. However, when your immune system is disrupted, it puts itself unnecessarily on constant defense, sending inflammation continually rippling throughout your body. In this state, it's working against you instead of for you by switching focus from the antigen it's supposed to attack, and instead launching a targeted strike on your own cells, tissues, or other harmless material.

What causes this disruption in our immune system that changes it from internal watchdog to worst enemy? It could be a number of things, any of which can come together in any combination to create the perfect storm.

COULD INFLAMMATION BE LURKING WITHIN YOU?

Maybe you have an existing autoimmune or other chronic disease. If that's the case, new research confirms that you very likely have a disruption of your digestive tract that is making it all too easy for harmful ingredients to enter your system, triggering or worsening inflammation.

Or maybe you don't have any existing known conditions, consider yourself healthy, and aren't aware of the cumulative effect of eating processed foods, more sugar than you think, a diet containing chemicals, additives, foods you are sensitive to, and exposure to environmental toxins. You just know that sometimes you feel like crap. Maybe you have mood swings, persistent headaches or infections, digestion upsets, skin irritations, or low energy levels and just accept it as a part of day-to-day life. Whether you realize it or not — these diet and lifestyle factors can create a toxic load on your system, and can trigger a shift from good health to poor.

Conditions Associated with Chronic Inflammation

- ADHD
- Allergies
- Alzheimer's disease
- Anxiety
- Asthma
- Autism
- Autoimmune disease (rheumatoid arthritis, Hashimoto's thyroiditis, multiple sclerosis, celiac disease, gout, type 1 diabetes, psoriasis, lupus, and more)
- Cancer
- Cardiovascular disease
- Dementia
- Depression
- Diabetes (Type 2)
- Eczema
- Endometriosis
- Fibromyalgia
- Infertility
- Inflammatory bowel disease (Crohn's disease, ulcerative colitis)
- Obesity

Chronic inflammation has the potential to light your whole damn body on fire. It can be destructive, and for some, downright deadly. It is critical that we understand what ignites the fire and take action to put out the flames.

CHAPTER 2:

DIGESTION AND DISEASE

Our digestive system is the foundation for wellness and immunity, having the highest concentration of immune cells in our entire body. It was Hippocrates who first said, "all disease begins in the gut." The guy has a pretty good reputation, so I don't take his proclamation lightly. And though this wise, founding father of medicine first realized this over 2,000 years ago, most people seem to be surprised to know that a digestion (or "gut") issue could be the culprit for a variety of symptoms outside of the expected gas, bloating and poop issues.

The gut has four quite critical functions:

1. To digest food and convert it into vitamins
2. To absorb nutrients
3. To prevent toxins and pathogens from entering the bloodstream
4. To activate thyroid hormones, which are involved in almost every physiological process in the body

A big determinant to ensuring the above processes work effectively and efficiently is the makeup of the bacteria, or microorganisms that live within the digestive tract, otherwise known as your gut microbiome.

INTRODUCTION TO THE MICROBIOME

Your microbiome is loosely defined as the community of microorganisms or microbes (beneficial and harmful) that share our body space — not only in our gut, but on our skin, in our mouths, noses, throats, lungs, and urinary tracts. The microbiome as a whole is the source of intense, ongoing research. And while researchers have not yet been able to correlate specific microbes with specific diseases, they have acknowledged:

"What is clear...is that the microbiome is probably an important factor in many diseases, a factor that has been neglected in the past."

The American Academy of Microbiology estimates that our bodies have almost three times the amount of bacteria making up our microbiome (about 100 *trillion*) than we do human cells in our entire body. But, don't let this fact cause concern (yet). While the harmful, pathogenic bacteria (e.g. coliform bacteria like *E. Coli,* yeasts, fungus, parasites) are the ones we have been so focused on in the past, most of the bugs, like lactobacillus and bifidobacter, are actually beneficial, or commensal, bacteria.

THE GUTS OF THE MATTER

While the microbiome as a whole is a fascinating and timely topic, we are going to stay focused on the micro demographic in our digestive system. Not only does our digestive system house about

70% of our immune cells, 95% of our serotonin and 90% of *all* neurotransmitters also take up residence there as well.

Ideally, we have a strong, working relationship with the friendly bugs.

Through our diet we provide the nutrients to feed these beneficial bacteria, and in turn, they keep our immunity in check, make certain vitamins, regulate our metabolism, and assist in gene expression, digestion, and many other processes that we are continuing to learn about.

It's a win/win. Or, at least it should be.

CATEGORIES OF DISRUPTION

Unfortunately, your digestive system and the related processes it is in charge of can be compromised via two general categories. (here's where we start to get concerned):

1. *Dysbiosis*

The goal for a healthy gut is to have the good, beneficial bacteria outweigh the bad. The good guys act as a physical barrier to the bad. If the good guys get killed off, don't show up in the first place, or if you consume a diet that feeds your body more bad bacteria, it makes more room for the bad (pathogenic) to take over. This leads the way to a skewed ratio of much more bad bugs to good, aka dysbiosis.

2. *Leaky Gut*

The protective lining of your digestive system or gut lumen (the space inside the tube of your intestine that regulates the passage of nutrient particles into your bloodstream), can be damaged by various diet and environmental factors. This causes your digestive system to become overly permeable. And when this protective barrier breaks down, it takes down your entire system with it.

Usually your intestinal wall is woven like a piece of cheesecloth. When it's "leaky" though, it's more like a tennis net. This series of openings allows larger, undigested nutrient particles to get into your bloodstream before they've had time to marinate in the proper digestive juices. Various toxins and bacteria can also pass through. These escapees are viewed as foreigners by your immune system and trigger an antibody reaction leading to inflammation, putting a huge strain on your entire system.

Several years ago, leaky gut was only truly acknowledged in more alternative settings, but with new research available identifying how the gut lining breaks down and its association with inflammation, autoimmune disease, cancer and other chronic conditions, it is becoming more widely accepted. Today, you will hear leaky gut referred to as "intestinal hyperpermeability" or a "disrupted microbiome".

The words "leaky" and "gut" aren't painting a very pretty picture but the concept is imperative to almost everything we'll discuss. If your gut health isn't on point, your overall health won't be either. Getting off course compromises your immunity (e.g. inappropriate inflammatory responses), detoxification process (your ability to deal with toxins in the environment), nutrient status, and neurotransmitter balance. In fact, the health of your gut even plays a role in determining how your genetic dispositions will manifest.

CHAPTER 3:

THE INTERPLAY OF YOUR CELLS, YOUR GENES, YOUR ENVIRONMENT AND YOUR GUT

There is a strong interrelationship between how our cells function, how our genes are expressed, our environment, our microbiome, inflammation and chronic disease.

Cells — trillions of them — are the building blocks of each and every one of us as living organisms. What keeps our cells functioning appropriately (i.e. preventing disease) is providing them with the proper nutrients and avoiding insults from toxins in our environment. Our cells also contain our individual genetic makeup, or DNA.

We are all individuals, made up of unique sets of genes and characteristics. What makes each of us even more distinctive is that our diet, lifestyle and environment can combine to determine whether our genes manifest into good health or poor. To some degree, we're able to choose to create a body that is either disease resistant or inflammation prone.

YOUR GENES ARE NOT THE COMPLETE PICTURE

What may be surprising is that for most chronic disease, your genes only make up 10–20% of your risk. What makes up the other 80–90%? Your environment — what you are putting in, on and around your body. As Chris Kresser, M.S., L.Ac, a global leader in functional and integrative medicine so brilliantly states:

"Genes may load the gun, but environment pulls the trigger."

Think of our health like undeveloped film, and the process in which it's turned into a photo. Every aspect could influence what the end result is — the developing chemicals, processes, camera, and photographer. Each factor has the ability to make up for, or sabotage one another.

Similarly, our genes, environment, diet and lifestyle are all powerful influencers determining the status of our health. The amount of toxins we are exposed to through our food and the products that go on and around our bodies, our ability to adequately eliminate those toxins, the nutrient deficiencies we may have and other stressors our bodies might endure all determine how our picture of health develops.

So no matter what you're starting with, ask yourself how you would like your photo to turn out.

There are now dedicated fields of study (epigenetics, nutrigenomics) that look specifically at how these external factors determine whether your genes will manifest into disease. And we now know much more about specific genetic variations that can compromise your ability to absorb and process critical nutrients and detoxify from chemicals and toxins you are exposed to in the environment. These variations can be tested for (rather inexpensively) and addressed with targeted supplementation to address nutrient deficiencies that can lead to disease.

GUT MICROBIOME AND GENETIC EXPRESSION

Because our gut microbiome plays a critical role in regulating our immune response, detoxification processes and nutrient status, one of the biggest factors affected by your environment — and the effect our environment will have on our genes — is the gut microbiome. Research has recently identified that the key determinant in allowing environmental factors to trigger faulty genes is having a leaky gut. When leaky gut combines with environmental insults (toxins from the environment, nutrient deficiencies) it acts as an alarm, waking those genes and allowing the predispositions to manifest.

The association of leaky gut and disease is especially strong with autoimmune conditions, but it is also associated with many other conditions, including:

- Allergies & food sensitivities
- Alcoholism
- Autism
- Cardiac conditions
- Childhood hyperactivity
- Diabetes
- Inflammatory bowel disease (including Crohn's & ulcerative colitis) & other digestive issues
- Obesity
- Mood/cognitive disorders
- Skin conditions (acne, psoriasis, eczema, rashes)

Compounding the issue, having a leaky gut means your primary immunity protective barrier is down, making you even more susceptible to harm from your environment (pathogens, toxins, undigested food particles) and further inflammation.

PART TWO
IGNITION

CHAPTER 4:

FOOD: HOW WE'VE LOST OUR WAY

When we focus on nutrition, for the most part we think of fast energy and satisfying hunger. But let's think of food as a healing, nurturing part of life for a minute. Food isn't just calories, carbs and a quick fix — it's medicine, and whether you're in the throes of a catastrophic health crisis or not, it's time to consider the healing power it holds.

Every time we eat, we are either feeding our good health, or we're feeding our latent potential for disease. The trillions of cells we are made up of require specific nutrients to function properly (i.e. prevent disease). Nutrients allow your body to make energy, build and maintain tissues, and regulate bodily processes. Nutrients are also what make up the building blocks of our biochemistry. To ignore the power of our diet is dismissive. And yet, we do dismiss it, day after day, assuming we can just fix things on the other end with medications.

A PARADIGM SHIFT

Conventional theory has taught us to believe that eating healthy means counting calories, carbs, and fat grams, when what we should really be focused on is food quality, balance, and food sensitivities. If this is your first venture into the clean eating, anti-inflammatory movement, this is your chance to refocus on the bigger picture—and get back to common sense in many ways. Merely looking at numbers has primed today's standard American diet (SAD) to be inflammatory. It's time to put away the calculators. And it's definitely time to stop buying and consuming over-processed, bastardized versions of food in a misguided attempt to eradicate everything we've been told is "bad" from our diets.

An anti-inflammatory diet is more about the *quality* of the food we put into our bodies, and less about a limited *quantity*. For some people, this can be a hard-to-grasp shift from a widely accepted paradigm. With calories, fat grams, scales, and calculators, things are in our control — or so we think — and we like that. Evidence proving that the quality of our food affects our health (and our waistline) exists in abundance. But shifting perspective away from the numbers game can still seem like a leap of faith. We need to start thinking in terms of what kinds of foods motivate our bodies to work well for us. What are the nutrients in that food that are going to help our systems prevent inflammation? Likewise, what's in our food that's going to piss off our bodies and set them ablaze?

FOOD QUALITY – WHAT IT REALLY MEANS

What does the term "food quality" mean to you? Is it about the beautiful presentation of your meal? How far in advance you had to book a reservation for the exclusive restaurant with the celebrity chef? Or are you simply satisfied if your food hasn't landed on the floor before finding its way to your plate?

Decades ago, humans all ate organic food, and cows and other livestock were grass-fed because they lived outside in the pasture. But over the years things like mass production and profit margins have changed the way our food is produced. These days, organic food isn't the norm, it's a specialty item that we have to seek out. And while a popular topic — both in nutrition and politics — you won't find any formal, governmental recommendation on the quality of the sources of our food to help guide you. There is now more to avoid in our quest for whole foods and more to think about when we consider the quality of our food.

Note: Examining the social, environmental, and ethical perspectives on what we eat, where it's sourced, and how it's produced could be a book (or five) in itself. Because this book shines a spotlight on inflammation and disease, we will focus here on the related issues with the most evidence behind them. This information may concern you, and it should. But don't allow it to consume you with worry. The step-by-step solutions in Part Three will provide you with the tools — and the confidence — you need to make changes.

PESTICIDES AND GMOS

BACKGROUND

These are no doubt two topics you hear about daily. Maybe even hourly. But do you really understand the back story and why they are so harmful to your health? They are separate, yet related issues.

- Pesticides are substances used to kill, repel, or control certain forms of plant or animal life that are considered to be pests. They can include herbicides (for weeds), insecticides (for insects), fungicides (for molds/mildew), and disinfectants (for bacteria).

- Genetically-modified organisms (GMOs) are organisms whose genetic material has been artificially manipulated through genetic engineering in a laboratory producing unstable combinations of plant, animal, bacteria, and viral genes that do not occur naturally. This allows them to withstand larger amounts of the pesticides mentioned above.

- Twenty-six countries have banned the use of GMO crops and 64 others — including 28 nations in the European Union, Japan, Australia, Brazil, Russia and China — require the labeling of GMOs. However, the U.S. has not banned them, nor have we implemented any laws to require labeling. In fact, 80% of all conventional processed food in the U.S. contains GMOs.

- The most commonly genetically-modified crops are soy and corn. As of 2015, per the USDA, 94% of soy and 89% of corn is made from genetically modified crops. Guides on all genetically modified crops, as well as the most pesticide-heavy foods appear in the Toolkit.

ROLE IN INFLAMMATION AND DISEASE

- Many pesticides are known as estrogenic, meaning they can mimic the effect of estrogen, disrupting the action of our own hormones. These are known as endocrine disruptors. This will be covered in detail in Chapter 6, but for now know that this class of toxins plays a key role in fertility issues and contributes to the disruption of your microbiome (leaky gut).

- Pesticides — in particular the herbicide glyphosate — have been linked to non-Hodgkin's lymphoma as well as many other health conditions. Children are particularly susceptible to adverse effects, including neurodevelopment issues.

- Because GMO crops have the ability to withstand larger amounts of pesticides, the health concerns are heightened because of the sheer volume of the chemicals applied.

- Genetically-modified crops have been linked with severe liver and kidney damage, disturbance to pituitary gland function (an endocrine gland releasing many hormones, including your thyroid hormones), increased rates of large tumors and premature deaths.

- Genetically-modified crops produce a Bt *(Bacillus thuringienesis)* toxin that has been shown to alter immune function and increase gut permeability.

FACTORY-RAISED ANIMALS

BACKGROUND

For a well-nourished, healthy body, you need to consume well-nourished, healthy animals. Unfortunately, unless you are taking careful measures to ensure consumption of high-quality meat and fish that isn't always the case. It's a simple supply chain issue.

- Conventional livestock (i.e. not organic or grass-fed or pastured/pasture-raised) are no longer roaming the hills nibbling on inflammation-fighting grass. They are raised in confined animal feeding operations, or "CAFO"s — with no room to roam, and fed a diet of pesticide-laden, genetically-modified corn.

- We have an excess of this microbiome-disrupting corn (thanks to Farm Bills that provide subsidies to farmers who overgrow it) with 60% being used to feed CAFO livestock. A diet of corn (instead of grass) speeds up weight gain and shortens their lifespan (which gets them to slaughter earlier), and all that means one thing: money.

- Cows are not built to digest corn. They are ruminants, which are meant to digest grass. When a cow is introduced to corn it disturbs their digestion, causing them to get sick. Because of this, they are given their first course of antibiotics. And more courses will likely follow due to poor health from their feed and their overcrowded living conditions.

- Rather than being caught in its natural, wild environment, much of our fish (approximately half of our salmon) is now raised in fish farms, or aquacultures, where they receive contaminated fish food containing carcinogenic polychlorinated biphenyls, or PCBs.

- Farmed salmon is also fattened, similar to cows. And because PCBs are stored in the fat tissues, farmed salmon can contain five to 10 times the amount of PCBs than that of wild.

- Certain fish can contain very high levels of the heavy metal mercury, including king mackerel, marlin, shark, swordfish, tile fish, and orange roughy.

ROLE IN INFLAMMATION AND DISEASE

- Of the 24 million pounds of microbiome-altering antibiotics produced each year in the U.S., 19 million of it is fed to our factory-farmed livestock. When we consume these animals, we ingest those antibiotics as well, which then kills off our own beneficial bacteria and leads to a disrupted microbiome, or leaky gut.

- CAFO livestock are given synthetic growth hormones and steroids which drastically boosts production, but contributes to our altered digestion and inflammation in the process.

- There is a nutritional opportunity cost. With CAFO animals not grazing on grass (where the terms "grass-fed" and "pastured" come from), they are severely deficient in anti-inflammatory nutrients. Meat from beef, bison, lamb and goats that have been grass-fed has been found to have:

- two to four times the amount of omega-3 fatty acids
- three to five times the amount of conjugated linoleic acid (CLA)
- more vitamin E, beta-carotene, vitamin C, and significantly more of the fat-soluble vitamins A and D, which play a critical role in maintaining your immune system.

- The PCBs in farmed salmon are five to 10 times the amount of carcinogenic PCBs than that of wild. Farmed salmon has also been shown to contain significantly higher levels of several other chemical contaminants, including brominated flame retardants, pesticides (including DDT) and carcinogenic polynuclear aromatic hydrocarbons, or PAHs.

CAFO Animals and Depression

The grass consumed by grass-fed/pastured livestock is much higher in the essential amino acid tryptophan, than the grains (primarily corn) that CAFO animals feed on. Tryptophan is the precursor to the neurotransmitter serotonin associated with our mood. Low serotonin and chronic inflammation are both associated with depression.

FOOD ADDITIVES

We've discussed how the quality of fresh produce and animal products can be compromised. But when you purchase conventional packaged foods, you have even less control over what's in that bag. Besides simply displacing more nutrient-dense, anti-inflammatory whole foods, they are all too often made with a variety of synthetic chemicals that further trigger damage to our microbiome, and contribute to inflammation.

There are more than 10,000 additives in our food supply that have never been proven safe by the FDA, entering our food system by a loophole classification referred to as GRAS (Generally Recognized as Safe). Regularly ingesting these ingredients, which are seen as toxins to your body, causes free radical damage (read: premature aging of cells), hampers the immune system, and can even be carcinogenic.

Let's talk about those that are most cause for concern.

FOOD DYES

- Food dyes are found in almost any type of conventional packaged product available — candy, frostings, commercial cereals, yogurt, juices, condiments, packaged mac and cheese, and the list goes on. Sometimes they are even used in fresh fruit and fish.
- Our individual daily consumption has gone up over five times in the last 50+ years.
- Previously made from coal tar, they are now made from petroleum (i.e. gasoline)
- Food dyes have been shown to be carcinogenic, cause allergies, and promote hyperactivity.
- Many food dyes have already been banned from the food supply due to adverse health effects when studied in lab animals; however, many remain.
- Look for them listed in the ingredient list as:

• Blue 1	• Red 3
• Blue 2	• Red 40
• Citrus Red 2	• Yellow 5
• Green 3	• Yellow 6
• Orange B	• FD&C (followed by any color)

PROPYL PARABEN

- Found in food dyes and foods like certain packaged tortillas and pastries, propyl paraben is used as a preservative.
- It acts as a synthetic estrogen and has been associated with accelerating the growth of breast cancer cells.
- Propyl paraben has been found to decrease sperm counts in rats given doses within the FDA's approved limits and in a study from Harvard, it was linked to impaired fertility in women.

ARTIFICIAL AND NATURAL FLAVORS

- Countering intuition, these two aren't that different from a chemistry perspective. To be considered a "natural" flavor, it simply has to be derived from some type of plant.
- Both artificial and natural flavors are made up of 80–90% solvents (including propylene glycol), emulsifiers, flavor modifiers, and preservatives.

BHA AND BHT

- Butylated hydroxyanisole (BHA) and butylated hydroxytoluene (BHT) are petroleum-derived preservatives and stabilizers that can illicit an allergic reaction in some people and can trigger hyperactivity.

- Often, they are included to create an addiction to the food so that you consume more.

- There are concerns of them being carcinogenic and estrogenic.

MONOSODIUM GLUTAMATE (MSG)

- Considered a flavor enhancer, MSG is made of a sodium salt from the amino acid glutamic acid.

- It is on the list of additives needing further study by the FDA for being mutagenic (a chemical agent that alters your genes, including those that can cause cancer), teratogenic (causing birth defects), and causing reproductive effects.

- It has been shown to cause brain damage in multiple animal studies and has been linked to the following adverse effects: obesity, eye damage, headaches, fatigue and disorientation, depression, rapid heartbeat, tingling, and numbness.

NITRATES & NITRITES

- Nitrates can be either sodium or potassium nitrate and are used as preservatives and color fixatives in cured meats (e.g. hot dogs, deli meats, bacon).

- Specifically, nitrates have been associated with stomach, esophageal, brain, and thyroid cancers.

- Though no causal link has been confirmed, the World Health Organization's International Agency for Research on Cancer (IARC) has declared that ingested nitrites and nitrates are likely to be human carcinogens.

POTASSIUM BROMATE

- Here in the U.S., due to industrial baking practices (during which dough isn't left to rise naturally in open air), potassium bromate is used to expedite the rising process, as well as to strengthen bread and cracker dough.

- It has been labeled as a Category 2B carcinogen by the IARC and it is banned throughout the European Union, Canada, Nigeria, Brazil, Peru and China.

- While baking converts most potassium bromate to non-carcinogenic potassium bromide, research has shown that bromate residues are still detectable in finished bread in small but significant amounts.

- Potassium bromate is toxic to your kidneys and can damage your DNA. In animal studies, it causes tumors in multiple sites. It is listed as a known carcinogen by the state of California, but the U.S. still allows it to be added to flour.

ALUMINUM

- Aluminum can be found in food additives like sodium aluminum phosphate and sodium aluminum sulfate. It can also occur in conventional table salt and unpurified water.

- Other forms of aluminum can be found in the environment, medications, and certain vaccines.

- Excess aluminum has been associated with developmental and neurological effects, including neurotoxicity.
- It has been associated with an abnormal immune response related to various disease states, especially autoimmune disease, and a disrupted microbiome.

PROCESSED SWEETENERS

Refined sugar has been robbed of all the vitamins, minerals, proteins, enzymes, and other beneficial nutrients that original sugar cane or beet contains. Not only is it devoid of any nutritional value, it can actually cause your body to utilize its own supplies of certain micronutrients like calcium, potassium, thiamin, and chromium.

And when sweeteners have been over processed and are as pervasive as the products listed below, a whole host of other problems occur.

HIGH FRUCTOSE CORN SYRUP (HFCS)

- High fructose corn syrup is a liquid, processed sweetener made by corn refiners. Corn is combined with sodium hydroxide, hydrochloric acid and certain enzymes resulting in a chemical compound that contains heavy metal contaminants, like mercury.
- It is found in many products including baked goods, granola bars, cereal, juice and soda, and many condiments.
- Unlike regular cane sugar (sucrose), fructose from HFCS does not require digestion so it goes straight into the liver and is rapidly absorbed into the bloodstream causing a spike in inflammatory insulin, triggering the production of triglycerides and harmful types of cholesterol leading to a condition known as fatty liver.

- High fructose corn syrup is associated with diabetes, heart disease, cancer, and more. It also depletes the mechanism that maintains the integrity of your intestinal lining, (i.e. keeps your gut from being leaky).

ARTIFICIAL SWEETENERS

- Artificial sweeteners include aspartame, acesulfame, sucralose, sugar alcohols such as maltitol and xylitol, and the newly approved advantame (a derivative of aspartame).

- Artificial sweeteners can inhibit your natural production of serotonin, contributing to depression. And despite their lack of calories, the sweetness still raises your blood sugar, increasing inflammatory insulin levels. They are also extremely addictive.

- Aspartame is about two hundred times sweeter than sugar and is used in more than 6,000 products worldwide. And while concern over its role in various cancers (including brain, bladder, stomach, lymphoma and leukemia, breast, pancreatic, stomach, colon and endometrial) has largely been dismissed, it receives more complaints for adverse health effects than any other additive.

- Common complaints of aspartame include headaches, stomach irritation, insomnia, seizures, urinary tract infections, and neurological and behavioral disturbances. It has also been found to compromise metabolism, genetic material, nerve function, and hormone balance.

- Sucralose — at consumption levels that are approved by the FDA — suppresses beneficial gut bacteria, including acidophilus and bifidobacter, contributing to dysbiosis and a leaky gut.

Times have changed and so has our food. The onus is now on us as consumers to read the fine print and prioritize better quality ingredients — and better health.

CHAPTER 5:

OUT OF BALANCE: CARBOHYDRATES, FAT, PROTEIN, SUGAR, ANTIOXIDANTS

Clearing the unnecessary synthetic chemicals out of our diet is a critical step towards reducing inflammation. But just as important is getting the correct balance of nutrients going in. Old guidelines and paradigms taught us principles like limiting fats and making grains and other carbohydrates the mainstay of our diets. Even though these guidelines have been dismissed with current research, the messaging is still so pervasive, I find that most people — including the mainstream media — can't let it go.

So here and now, I will ask you to do yourself a gigantic favor: forget everything you knew about what "good" and "bad" foods are. Open your mind to a new set of rules, grounded in current research (and some common sense), that will help put out the flames of inflammation.

WE NEED MORE (OF THE RIGHT KIND OF) FAT

It was 1980 when the "Dietary Guidelines for Americans" were published, and policy started to focus on limiting total fat to 30% or less of our calories. What followed was an onslaught of low-fat and fat-free products, marketing, and messaging that is still very much in play today, making it one of the most difficult paradigms to change.

What got lost is that fat is an essential part of our diet. It aids in brain and eye development (the brain itself is made up of 60% fat), regulates blood sugar, promotes tissue healing and proper immune function, and is critical for vitamin D synthesis (a deficiency is very common in chronic disease). Fat is also the vehicle that carries and delivers fat-soluble vitamins (A, D, E, K) and nutrients like phytonutrients (believed to play a role in cancer prevention and serve as anti-inflammatories) to your body. This is why not consuming enough fat could result in various skin symptoms, brittle nails, aching joints, depression, ADHD, diabetes, weight GAIN, and even cancer.

We need to eat more fat, and we need to balance the types of fats that we eat. The key is to focus on oils and fats that are pesticide- and GMO-free and minimally processed (e.g. extra-virgin and expeller-pressed) instead of consuming chemically-processed, possibly genetically-modified, unstable (i.e. oxidized, which is damaging to your cells) fats like canola, corn, soy, or vegetable oil, or partially-hydrogenated margarines that are found in most processed foods. This eliminates the use of toxic chemicals and helps the fats retain their vital nutrients and delicate flavors.

BALANCING OMEGA-3 AND OMEGA-6 FATS

Balancing the kinds of fats we eat is just as important as eating the right amount of it. Omega-6 fats can come from healthy sources like seeds, nuts, and beans. A small amount is essential. But if we go in the other direction and consume large, concentrated amounts, the positive effect turns into a negative and inflammation can actually be created. Historically, American diets used to be close to a ratio of 1:1 of omega-6 to omega-3 fats. But with our current standard American diet (SAD), the balance is way off, currently estimated at 15 (omega 6): 1 (omega-3).

And it is this skewed RATIO — not the TOTAL fat — that is causing the inflammation that can lead to chronic health conditions such as cancer, heart disease, and autoimmune disease.

ANTI-INFLAMMATORY OMEGA-3 FAT SOURCES:

- wild, fatty fish (like salmon)
- grass-fed or pastured animal products
- chia seeds, flax seeds

GOOD OMEGA-6 FAT SOURCES TO INCLUDE:

- extra-virgin and expeller-pressed olive oil
- avocado

- whole seeds and nuts
- wild, grass-fed or pasture-raised animal fats

OMEGA-6 FATS SOURCES TO AVOID:

- processed vegetable and other oils: canola, corn, soy, peanut
- partially hydrogenated margarines
- animal fats from CAFO (corn-fed) animals

SATURATED FAT IS NOT THE ENEMY

Saturated simply means that the fat is complete in the molecular structure, giving them stability (this is why they don't oxidize). And saturated fats play important roles in our health — like protecting our cell walls, keeping blood sugar in check, and getting us those fat-soluble vitamins (A, D, E, K) and calcium I mentioned above. Butter in particular is very nutrient-dense, containing multiple vitamins and minerals — it's an especially good source of vitamin A, 18 amino acids and eleven different kinds of fat. One such fat, conjugated linoleic acid, has been shown to have beneficial effects on a range of inflammatory conditions. Another fat, butyrate, is an essential fatty acid for brain health, and has been shown to specifically suppress inflammation in the gut.

Before the 1930's, processed vegetable oils weren't used because traditional — and saturated — fats like butter and cream, were preferred. Coconut and palm oil (more saturated fats) were also used commonly used back then. And guess what — our rates of heart disease, cancer, and depression were much lower then.

It was twenty years later, around 1950, that events led to the medical community flipping the switch on the use of saturated fats and this intensified in the 1980's. They became convinced that saturated fat in butter could cause heart disease, and that the polyunsaturated fat in vegetable oil and margarine was beneficial to your heart. And we quickly saw policy — and our pantries — follow suit. However, another 60+ years later, we have multiple studies that have shown that saturated fats do not play a role in coronary death. Because they burn at such a steady and reliable pace, they are actually the preferred energy source for your heart. Multiple studies have also shown that a higher-saturated-fat, lower-carbohydrate diet resulted in improved cholesterol and insulin levels, reduced weight and is not related to increased cardiovascular risk.

GOOD SOURCES OF SATURATED FAT:

- coconut oil
- palm oil
- animal fat from organic, wild or pastured animals

A complete guide to which fats to use, and when, is included in the Toolkit.

WE NEED LESS (OF THE WRONG TYPE OF) CARBOHYDRATES

Before we get started, let me be clear: By no means am I about to talk about a low-carb or Atkins-esque diet plan. I am not going to tell you to stop eating fruit or to start counting the grams of carbs in the nuts you eat (I am actually pretty averse to doing any counting at all). The carbohydrates I am referring to are grains, most specifically refined grains and starches.

The classic Food Guide Pyramid carried a small bit of fats and oils at the tip top, and the sturdy base was built on a foundation of carbohydrates from grains and starches. Up to 60% of our calories, in fact. This has since been replaced with revised guidelines and we know now that it is in fact a diet high in refined carbohydrates that is linked to coronary heart disease and many other chronic conditions. But day after day — in the media and on people's plates — I still see this preference to carbohydrates held on to as the norm.

THE REAL STORY ON GRAINS

While whole grains have always been encouraged in government recommendations, that definition is used loosely. Today, having the term whole grain on label does not have a clear definition. It can allow for a portion of the product to be refined (stripped of their nutrient-dense, fiber-rich bran and germ). Refined grains and starches — which accounts for most of the grain consumed in the U.S. — spike insulin levels creating inflammation, poor cognitive function, poor blood sugar management, fat storage and fatigue.

True, 100% whole grains — in appropriate amounts — can be part of a healthful diet, providing B vitamins, fiber and prebiotics (nutrients that the beneficial probiotics feed off of). But beware, they should not be the mainstay of our diets. And for some, they can be quite problematic. Grains contain properties including: oxalates, phytates, lectins, and saponins, which bind to minerals, preventing absorption and inhibiting digestive enzymes.

A general recommendation would be to have grains be approximately 25% of your meals. However, depending on your condition, you may need to avoid all grains for a period of time. We can get the carbohydrates, fiber, and B vitamins we need for energy from whole fruits and vegetables, root vegetables and legumes (lentils, chickpeas, and beans). Soaking or fermenting all grains, beans and seeds prior to cooking them is ideal to help ensure complete digestion.

Who Should Avoid Grains?

If you have serious digestive issues, especially if any type of painful bloating is involved, you have been diagnosed with conditions such as small intestinal bacterial overgrowth (SIBO), you are having acute flare-ups with inflammatory bowel disease (Crohn's disease or ulcerative colitis), or you have severe autoimmune disease, a grain-free diet is recommended for a period of time to prevent further damage and allow your gut to heal. It is always recommended that you work with a professional health practitioner to address the underlying issues and ensure your diet is otherwise balanced. A concern would be that consumption of carbohydrates, fiber and B vitamins could get too low. Root vegetables (e.g. yams or sweet potatoes) are good replacements to address all three nutrients.

LEAKY GUT & GLUTEN

If grains contain gluten (wheat, rye, barley, spelt — almost any conventional flour or grain you will come by unless specifically marketed otherwise), they are even more of an issue when you have inflammatory conditions or a disrupted microbiome. Undigested gluten can be a premature escapee from your digestive system and seen as a foreign invader, inappropriately triggering the immune response. In addition, consuming gluten releases a protein (zonulin) that loosens up the tight junctions of your digestive system — or opens the spaces of your intestinal lining. In those susceptible, this can lead to a leaky gut (more about this in Chapter 6).

WE NEED LESS SUGAR

Americans consume on average, 130 pounds of sugar every year. This is due not only to the obvious sugar-laden desserts and sodas, but also due to the pervasiveness of added sugars to packaged foods. So, even when you mean well, and are trying to eat "healthy" — your granola bars, cereals...even your bottled salad dressing likely has sugars added to it. This is designed to not only make them more appetizing, but to get you to keep coming back for more. Sugar has been found to be as addictive as cocaine. And we build up a tolerance just like we would for any other drug.

HOW SUGAR ACTS IN YOUR BODY

Calories from sugar are metabolized differently than other foods. Sugar metabolism, especially in the case of processed fructose, can result in the attack of nerve endings and a fatty liver — contributing to strokes, diabetes, hypertension, and possibly dementia and cancer. It disrupts mineral and enzyme function, which not only can initiate new or worsen existing food sensitivities, but leads to toxicity and inflammation in various organs and tissues of the entire body.

Consumed refined sugar and other refined carbohydrates are absorbed very quickly causing a surge in glucose levels (also referred to as having a high Glycemic Index). This requires your pancreas to release a responding level of insulin to combat the high levels of glucose which are toxic to the body. Prolonged levels of elevated insulin contribute to inflammation. And, according to Dr. Louis C. Cantley, a researcher at Harvard/Beth Israel Deaconess, a high spike in insulin is a catalyst to certain cancers. One-third of cancers have insulin receptors (including breast and colon cancers) and the sugar (or glucose) helps the tumors to grow.

As with all refined carbohydrates, sugar feeds the pathogenic bacteria (e.g. yeast), allowing them to overtake the beneficial bacteria, leading to a disrupted microbiome, AKA leaky gut.

Ideally, all forms of sugar should be reduced as much as possible — but natural forms (like raw honey or black strap molasses) are safer and can provide other health benefits. Look for the guide on pantry staples in the Toolkit.

WE NEED MORE (OR LESS) ANIMAL PROTEIN

No doubt, eating meat is a polarizing issue, and the debate around the social and environmental concerns is beyond the scope of this book. I will instead stay focused on the nutrition, and the role high-quality meats play in an anti-inflammatory diet.

A common trend: people eat far too much animal protein (usually at the cost of important antioxidant-filled vegetables) or because of the fear and confusion around consuming animal products, avoid it altogether.

Consuming high-quality animal protein sources provides the right types of omega-6 fats and the anti-inflammatory omega-3 fats, and ensures you will be getting all of the essential amino acids — the building blocks of protein — in the most bioavailable (i.e. absorbable) form. Protein is critical for tissue growth and repair, enzymes and detoxification, and is especially important for healing permeability of the gut. If you've been hearing a lot about bone broths lately, this is why. They can be a great, concentrated source of tissue healing nutrients. Food from animals also provides much needed cholesterol. Cholesterol received from your diet should not be feared, it is critical for many functions in the body, including protecting cell membranes, brain function and hormone production and does not elevate the bad cholesterol in your blood.

Previous claims that meat is harmful to your health can be misleading and biased. Concerns about animal protein would best be explained if we compared a diet made up primarily of high-quality meat (unprocessed, organic, wild, grass-fed or pastured) vs. one made up of CAFO, GMO, corn-fed meat. But, that comparison doesn't exist in the research. What does exist in much of the research is confounding lifestyle factors, or what are known as "healthy user bias." This means that subjects who are likely to implement a behavior that is perceived as healthy (e.g. limit red meat) are also more likely to implement other healthy behaviors like not smoking, limiting alcohol or exercising more — all of which could have more significant effects on their health outcomes than the study subject itself (e.g. meat intake). When these other behaviors are at play, the meat consumption alone — especially when there is no differentiation of its quality — cannot not be isolated as the cause of ill health.

TO MEAT OR NOT TO MEAT?

So taking all of the above into consideration, if the question is "to meat or not to meat?", the answer is somewhere in the middle. Everyone's specific needs for animal protein — and all protein — will be different based on your individual condition. But the goal is to strive for a "plant strong" diet, made up of abundant whole vegetables and fruits with smaller amounts of high-quality animal protein. Based on the concepts we learned in Chapter 4, this means organic, grass-fed, or pastured animal sources or wild (not farmed) fish, and limited amounts of processed meat (ensuring that what you do eat is without nitrates). And limit cooking meat at very high temperatures (e.g. barbequing) which can release carcinogenic amines. With regard to quantity, a general rule of thumb is that when you consume animal protein, have it only make up about ¼ of your meal. Without specifically measuring portions, think of it as a side dish, rather than the main course. And work in non-animal protein sources (e.g. nuts or nut butters, beans) for a meal every day, or a day every week. Balance doesn't always have to be achieved within 24 hours.

WE NEED MORE VEGETABLES

With inflammation, you aren't only playing defense, trying to avoid any possible food that might ignite the flames. You need to also be on the offensive, fighting inflammation head on with nutrient dense, anti-inflammatory foods.

Two of the best weapons we have are whole vegetables and fruits, but unfortunately, most people consume far less than they should. It is estimated that only 9–32% of Americans consume the government recommended five daily servings of fruits and vegetables per day. Keep in mind, this data includes *any* type of fruits and vegetables — so it includes less nutrient-dense products like white potatoes and iceberg lettuce. And with the depletion of our soil lowering the nutrient content of our food, five servings per day may no longer be adequate. This means that at least 68–91% of Americans are lacking essential vitamins, minerals, and phytonutrients — all of which act as anti-inflammatory antioxidants in our systems and direct our cells to perform as they should to prevent disease.

Free Radicals and Antioxidants: Why They're So Important

Antioxidants (i.e. preventing or repairing oxidation, or damage, to your cells) play a critical role in keeping free radicals in check. And free radicals are what lead to oxidative stress, which has been linked to many inflammatory conditions like cancer, heart disease, diabetes, and autoimmune diseases. The major antioxidants are vitamins A, C and E, beta-carotene, and lycopene found in plant foods — primarily vegetables and fruits.

Green leafy vegetables in particular are nutritional powerhouses, providing many essential vitamins and minerals, including vitamin E (a potent inflammation-fighter), B vitamins, disease-fighting phytonutrients, and calcium.

All of this is to say that vegetables and fruits need to be a critical part — and the biggest part — of your diet. Research has shown that adequate consumption of fruits and vegetables is a key nutritional indicator of chronic disease risk (regardless of being a meat eater or a vegetarian). If our goal is to have 25% grains and 25% meat on our plates (with at least one ample serving of fat), the other 50% of your meal should be fresh vegetables and fruit (mostly vegetables). Try to get five to seven servings per day. Your body will thank you.

CHAPTER 6:

GLUTEN, DAIRY AND OTHER FOOD SENSITIVITIES: THE COMPLETE STORY

A whole, balanced diet is critical, but addressing and eliminating foods sensitivities—which have the ability to consistently trigger your immune system—is one of the most critical steps you can take in reducing inflammation. Let's take a closer look and understand exactly what a food sensitivity is, what the most common ones are, and how to test for and remove them from your diet, healthfully.

FOOD SENSITIVITIES DEFINED

A food sensitivity is an immune-based, inflammatory reaction to a protein in a particular food (like the gluten protein in wheat, rye or barley, or the casein protein in milk products). When you consume a food you are sensitive to, your immune system creates an overabundance of IgG (immunoglobulin G) antibodies, which bind directly to the food as it enters the bloodstream.

This immune reaction can be delayed, which is why it is also commonly referred to as a delayed hypersensitivity. Reactions can appear anywhere from a couple of hours to several days after consumption. Most people don't even realize they have sensitivities to such foods because symptoms can be so elusive. But, regularly consuming foods that your body reacts to, even slightly, can put you in a constant state of inflammation.

Symptoms of food sensitivity:

- A strong craving for particular foods (especially with gluten and casein)
- Pain: headaches, stomach pain, joint pain and others
- Mood and cognitive issues: depression, anxiety, hyperactivity, foggy thinking
- Digestion issues: bloating, diarrhea, constipation, heartburn
- Skin upsets: acne, eczema, psoriasis, rashes

Most common food sensitivities:

- Gluten
- Dairy (casein)
- Soy
- Corn
- Eggs
- Yeast (including fermented products like vinegar)
- Nightshade vegetables (tomatoes, bell peppers, potatoes, eggplant)
- Citrus fruits
- Food additives

Gluten and casein warrant a deep dive here and are the two most common sensitivities. Due to their specific proteins and the way they are processed, they are the most problematic with regard to gut health and inflammation, and they are most closely correlated with specific chronic conditions.

Food Sensitivity vs. Food Allergy

While food allergies *could* be a result of issues with your gut microbiome (aka leaky gut) and inflammation, true food allergies are not the focus of this book.

Unlike a sensitivity, a food allergy results in an immediate hypersensitivity reaction, caused by histamines released after exposure. The severity of the reaction can range from hives to anaphylaxis—a potentially life-threatening condition that can cause the airways to close. A true food allergy is common in kids, but rare in adults. The most common foods that people are allergic to include: peanuts, tree nuts (such as walnuts, pecans and almonds), fish, shellfish, milk, eggs, and soy products. A true wheat allergy is actually quite uncommon. Food allergies are tested with blood tests looking for IgE (Immunoglobulin E) antibodies or a skin prick test (SPT) that would be performed in the office of an allergist/immunologist.

THE GLUTEN DEBATE

"I'm gluten-free" is likely the most polarizing statement in the health community today. Progressive practitioners (and their clients) devoutly stand by the role gluten can play in inflammation and overall immunity, while conventional medicine dismisses its legitimacy and even condemns the "dangers" of a gluten-free diet outside of a confirmed diagnosis of celiac disease.

Mainstream media has dutifully played its role by jumping on the topic and constantly feeding us the hype, and then rejoicing in the opportunity to run a follow-up feature with the gluten-free tag as the villain. But as with most stories, there are three sides: His, hers, and the truth. And in this case, the truth lies somewhere in the middle.

For the most part, gluten's overexposure — and the awareness it brings — is positive. All press is good press — especially when it brings to light the fact that gluten is linked to over 50 different disease states.

Diseases and Conditions Associated with Gluten Sensitivity:

- Autoimmune disease
- Fibromyalgia
- Infertility
- Endometriosis
- Osteoporosis
- Fatigue
- Skin conditions (e.g. psoriasis, eczema)
- Digestive disease (e.g. irritable bowel disease)
- Mood and cognitive issues including ADHD, anxiety and depression
- Cancer
- Autism
- Epilepsy

It is estimated that about 1% of Americans have celiac disease (CD). But, for every one person with CD, there are an estimated six or seven people with non-celiac gluten sensitivity (NCGS). For this population, it has been shown that there is a 35–72% increased risk of death (primarily due to cancer, heart and respiratory disease, but other causes are at play here as well). Unfortunately, due to the lag in recognition by conventional medicine, it takes on average five physicians and 10–11 years to diagnose a gluten sensitivity and it is estimated that 99% of those with a gluten sensitivity still are not aware of it.

What is Celiac Disease?

Celiac disease (CD) is an autoimmune disease, which is an illness that occurs when the body tissues are attacked by its own immune system. With CD, antibodies produced in reaction to gluten consumption damage the intestinal villi (small, finger-like protrusions in the wall of your small intestine), whose job it is to absorb food and nutrients. With those important little villi down and out, the results can be malabsorption of food leading to GI distress (i.e. diarrhea), anemia, and sometimes, weight loss. The only current treatment for CD is eliminating gluten from your diet completely.

Celiac disease symptoms are not isolated to GI symptoms as historically believed. It has been found that for every one patient with celiac disease who has GI symptoms, there are eight patients that present with completely different issues.

Celiac is associated with many other autoimmune disorders, including RA, type 1 diabetes, lupus, Hashimoto's thyroiditis, alopecia areata (hair loss) and scleroderma, as well as non-autoimmune chronic diseases and disorders such as Down syndrome, fibromyalgia, and chronic fatigue syndrome. Left untreated (i.e. not committing to a 100% gluten-free diet for life), CD can lead to certain cancers (primarily of the small bowel, esophagus and some non-Hodgkin lymphomas), iron-deficiency anemia, early onset of osteoporosis, pancreatic and gallbladder insufficiency, and neurologic issues. Celiac is detected with a blood test (prior to taking gluten out of the diet) and confirmed with a small bowel biopsy.

GLUTEN: WHAT IT IS AND WHAT IT ISN'T

So what IS gluten, how do you avoid it, and why would you want to?

Let's start at the beginning.

All foods are made up of three macronutrients — carbohydrate, protein and fat. Gluten is the protein complex that exists in grains, namely wheat, rye, spelt, and barley.

Gluten is a very large protein and it is very difficult to digest. In fact, the human body doesn't completely digest gluten at all. Gluten provides structure and elasticity for baked goods, but there are many concerns with the way our conventional, gluten-containing grains are processed and harvested today that make them especially harmful. Linking back to Chapter 3, we're talking about the use of bromate for quick rising (a possible carcinogen) and glyphosate herbicides to expedite the harvesting process and increase the yield.

If your body is not completely breaking down gluten, protein peptides can form and act on opiate receptors in the brain, mimicking the effects of drugs like heroin or morphine, creating cravings and/or an addiction to more of the gluten-containing food.

Common sense would indicate (correctly) that this doesn't sound beneficial to anyone, but for some, it creates a whole world of hurt.

HOW GLUTEN CAUSES TROUBLE

For people with inflammatory, chronic conditions (autoimmune or otherwise) and a disruption in their microbiome, gluten is especially problematic, because their body will have a harder time digesting it. It sits there bored in the intestine for a minute, then before it has had enough time to marinate in the proper digestive juices, it sneaks out through the tennis net gut lining and starts stumbling around. Eventually — and unfortunately — it can get into the bloodstream, and set itself up in various systems within the body depending on the specific genetic predisposition. At this point, the undigested food particle is seen as a foreign invader and the always-at-the-ready immune system attacks, resulting in an inflammatory response.

Even if your microbiome is right as rain, you're not exempt, as consuming high amounts of gluten can lead to future problems. Remember, when anyone eats gluten, it causes the release of a protein called zonulin, which unzips the tight junctions that hold together a currently intact intestinal lining. That is, it can create a leaky gut.

Autoimmune Disorders & Gluten Sensitivity

In autoimmune disease, messages get crossed. When triggered by a foreign invader, the immune system gets confused and starts to attack its bodies' own tissues. Which specific tissues, or systems, get attacked depends on the genetic predisposition. For example, with rheumatoid arthritis, joints are attacked. With multiple sclerosis, the central nervous system is attacked, with Hashimoto's thyroiditis, the thyroid is attacked.

The conventional treatment for autoimmune disease is to suppress the immune system with drugs. However, a more progressive approach is to identify and eliminate the source that is triggering the immune system. One of the biggest triggers is food sensitivities, with gluten at the top of the list.

Autoimmune Disorders & Gluten Sensitivity Cont.

It has been shown that 48% of patients who have recently developed RA also have anti-gliadin antibodies (inflammation-causing antibodies produced by your body in response to consuming gluten). And gluten sensitivity has been linked to many other autoimmune diseases which now affect more than 24 million Americans, as well as many other conditions.

Gluten is no joke. And if you find you do have a sensitivity, and you want to feel better, gluten is likely something you will need to say farewell to forever. For those concerned with the conventional-minded headlines about the dangers of the gluten-free diet, I have a newsflash of my own: Wheat and gluten are not essential nutrients. We don't have to consume either as part of a healthy diet. There are approximately zero nutrients exclusive to gluten-containing grains that can't be found elsewhere.

For much more detail on gluten, refer to my four-part blog series: shellymalone.com/blog. A complete list of gluten resources—including grains with and without gluten, hidden sources, and substitutes—is available in the Toolkit.

DAIRY/CASEIN SENSITIVITY

Like wheat, dairy contains a large, hard-to-digest protein. In wheat, we know that protein is called gluten. In dairy, the protein is referred to as casein (dairy contains another protein, whey, but a sensitivity to that is much more unlikely). Similar to gluten, casein can also permeate your gut lining, causing inflammation and leading to (or perpetuating) a disrupted microbiome, or leaky gut.

And if you already have issues with gluten, you should know that it has been found that approximately 50% of people with a sensitivity to gluten have a sensitivity to casein as well. This is due to underlying issues with immunity, the gut microbiome, and the fact that the enzymes required to digest gluten and to digest casein are the same (DPPIV, to be specific). Along with gluten, dairy is something you should prepare yourself to give up for some time. At least the conventional, cow's milk dairy you know now.

Casein Sensitivity vs. Lactose Intolerance

Casein sensitivity and lactose intolerance are very different types of reactions to dairy. Lactose intolerance is the inability to digest the *carbohydrate* in milk — lactose — due to a lack of the enzyme lactase. Some people are born with a deficient amount, but everyone's lactase supply wanes as they age. Casein sensitivity is an inflammatory reaction to a particular *protein* in diary, casein. Although, they are different issues, they can sometimes occur at the same time due to a disrupted gut microbiome. In general, lactose intolerance is considered less severe than a casein sensitivity.

HOW DAIRY DISAPPOINTS

The majority of the cows we have in America today are not the same breed as they once were. And this has a big effect on the composition of the milk that is produced. Specifically, the type of casein today's cow produces is much different. To elaborate...we used to have more of the Jersey and Guernsey breed of cows which produced A2 beta-casein — the same type of casein produced in goat, sheep and buffalo milks. However, now the most commonly seen breed in the U.S. is the Holstein cow, which produces an A1 beta-casein. A1 beta-casein breaks into an opiate protein (BCM7) that produces damaging antibodies which are related to many health conditions—most specifically, celiac disease, diabetes, multiple sclerosis, other autoimmune diseases and autism.

Additionally, today's conventional processing turns milk into a derelict product. Pasteurization kills the active enzymes and live active cultures that allow your body to digest dairy properly and also decreases the absorption of many vital nutrients, including: fat-soluble nutrients (vitamins A, D, E, K), certain minerals (manganese, copper, and iron), vitamin C, vitamin B6 and vitamin A. And if the cows are not specifically grass-fed they are also lacking the inflammation-fighting omega-3 fats and conjugated linoleic acid (CLA).

Even milk that has the virtuous organic label is subject to this strip down. If it's pasteurized, it's as bankrupt as the non-organic variety. That said, if the dairy *isn't* organic, you are ingesting all of the damaging products given to the cows in an effort to drastically boost production—products like synthetic growth hormones, steroids, genetically modified corn, and antibiotics. As addressed in Chapter 4, all of these antibiotics, steroids, and genetically modified organisms (GMOs) are big contributors to the breakdown of our digestion, and therein our entire immune system.

Conditions Linked to Casein Sensitivity

- Autoimmune conditions (celiac disease, diabetes, multiple sclerosis, rheumatoid arthritis, autism and others)
- Depression
- Autism
- ADHD
- Constipation and other digestive conditions
- Skin conditions (e.g. acne, eczema)
- SIDS (sudden infant death syndrome)
- Some cancers (breast, prostate, testicular and ovarian)
- Congestion
- Generalized inflammation which can manifest in many forms from ear infections to more serious conditions

GETTING REQUIRED NUTRIENTS WITHOUT DAIRY

As recently as 2015, highly regarded studies have found that consuming high levels of calcium from milk or supplements — which has basically been preached to us since year one of our lives — doesn't strengthen our bones. To the contrary, it has been found that those who drank the most milk had the highest risk of bone fractures and early death. In fact, the consumption of milk can actually lead to heart disease and kidney stones by building up in our arteries and kidneys.

We can get all the calcium we need from green leafy vegetables like kale, mustard greens, collards, Swiss chard and broccoli. Some other good sources are sesame seeds, bone-in fish, sweet potatoes, blackstrap molasses, and figs. Cow's milk doesn't even break the top ten list of highest calcium-containing foods — it's number 14.

Vitamin D can be found in eggs (which do not contain casein), fatty fish (tuna, salmon, sardines), and sun exposure. Vitamin D supplements can also be taken, although it is always best to have blood levels tested prior to this and work with a practitioner for appropriate dosing.

SOY, NIGHTSHADES AND OTHER SENSITIVITIES

While gluten and casein are at the top of the list of inflammation-producing food sensitivities, it is worth mentioning a couple of others. Corn and soy are also common culprits that I recommended removing from your diet for a few reasons:

- Soy requires the same digestive enzymes as gluten and dairy (DPPIV), to be broken down. So if you are lacking in those enzymes, soy can also end up as an undigested foreign invader eliciting an attack by the immune system.

- Corn contains certain types of proteins similar to wheat, which make it difficult to be digested.

- If corn and soy are not specifically labeled organic or non-GMO, you can almost bet they are genetically modified and laced with pesticide.

- Modern soy has been shown to be pro-estrogenic, suppressing the thyroid, causing reproductive problems, and stimulating cancer cells.

Nightshade vegetables are another group of foods that could cause sensitivities, particularly in autoimmune disease. If your symptoms change with the weather, this could be an indication that eliminating nightshades could benefit you. Common symptoms include muscle pain and tightness, morning stiffness, poor healing, arthritis, insomnia, gallbladder problems, and heartburn.

Nightshade vegetables include: tomatoes, potatoes (NOT sweet potatoes or yams), eggplant, all peppers (including paprika), ground cherries, goji berries, ashwagandha (an herb, common in supplements for fatigue and brain fog), cape gooseberries, garden huckleberries.

What About FODMAPS?

If you've been in on the food sensitivity or food intolerance discussion, you've probably already heard about this class of fermentable carbohydrates. The term FODMAP stands for: Fermentable Oligosaccharides (fructans and galacto-oligosaccharides like onions, Brussels sprouts, wheat, legumes), Disaccharides (specifically the carbohydrate in milk, lactose), Monosaccharides (specifically the carbohydrate in fruit, fructose) and Polyols (sugar alcohols — sorbitol, mannitol, xylitol, and maltitol — also certain fruits and vegetables like apples and cauliflower). To put into simple terms, these are specific carbohydrates that feed the bacteria in your gut microbiome, ferment, and then create gas. They can also draw water into the colon, which can cause diarrhea for people who don't tolerate them. This is the case for those who have a disrupted microbiome, small intestinal bacterial overgrowth (SIBO), or other digestive concerns. If you have symptoms like gas, abdominal pain, diarrhea, or constipation, consider avoiding high FODMAP foods. A full list of FODMAP foods will be in the Toolkit.

FOOD SENSITIVITY TESTING

Several blood tests for gluten and other foods sensitivities are available through various laboratories, including IgG, IgA or IgM antibody testing.

These tests can be helpful and provide a good piece to the overall individual's health puzzle, but there are some limitations to the process, with false negative results (wherein you do have a sensitivity, but your test reads negative) being the biggest issue. The test may not be comprehensive enough in the type of antigens and protein fractions they look for or you could react differently to the raw form of the food (commonly used in testing) than you do to the cooked form. Testing can also be expensive and is not usually covered by insurance.

You may also have heard of (or endured the situation yourself) where a food sensitivity test is taken and sensitivities to a large number of seemingly innocuous foods from bananas to pepper show up. When this is seen, it usually indicates that the underlying issue is a leaky gut, showing any food that someone eats often as triggering an immune response.

So, the best way to test for a sensitivity is to *completely* eliminate the food in question from your diet (not even a single crumb or sip) for at least two weeks, ideally four to six weeks. This is commonly called an elimination diet. The best place to start is with gluten, casein, soy, and corn. See if your symptoms improve. If they do, it is best not to reincorporate — just avoid consuming it (especially with gluten). If after that your symptoms still do not improve, it may be worth eliminating all common food sensitivities listed at the beginning of the chapter. A guide to following an elimination diet is available at shellymalone.com/inflamed.

If you do pursue food sensitivity testing, it is imperative that you test *before* removing gluten or other sensitivities from your diet for the most accurate results.

WILL YOU EVER BE ABLE TO EAT THESE FOODS AGAIN?

With food sensitivities (other than to gluten), after a period of time of going without, and working to right your microbiome (ideally alongside a professional practitioner who can customize a treatment plan), you could very well begin to tolerate again.

A good example of this is dairy. A sensitivity to dairy, or casein, often falls on a spectrum. After you have done a complete elimination of dairy for four to six weeks, you can test back small amounts of more easily digested versions.

Start with raw (i.e. not pasteurized) goat or sheep milk. In raw form, it retains the enzymes that help with digestion (plus better nutritional quality) and because it's from a goat or sheep, it will ensure it has the A2, rather than inflammatory A1 beta-casein. If that is tolerated, you could try raw, organic, grass-fed (or pastured) cow's milk.

Grass-fed (or pastured) butter is also something better tolerated because it is almost completely fat—therefore very little protein (casein).

Digestive enzymes (DPPIV) can also be taken to help with digestion, when consuming gluten, dairy or soy in very small amounts. Note: DPPIV will not give you a digestive system made of steel. And if you have a confirmed gluten sensitivity, I would only utilize these in the case of avoiding reactions from cross-contamination that might be experienced from eating food you can't confirm doesn't contain gluten (i.e. in a restaurant). Continuing to consume gluten with a known sensitivity, even occasionally, will continue to re-light the fire of inflammation and it can take weeks to months to recover from an exposure.

CHAPTER 7:

TOXIC RELATIONSHIPS: THE PRODUCTS IN YOUR HOME AND THE STRESS IN YOUR BODY

No matter how simple and clean we try to live, we are all inundated with products. Not just what we put on our bodies (lotion, perfume, hair products, make-up, topical medicines and ointments, etc.) but what is around us — both purposely and inadvertently. Think about what you spray your counter with when you clean. The candles you light and the air fresheners you use. The fumes you breathe in from certain chemicals in your furniture and other household materials. Some of the most seemingly benign products could be having big systemic effects on your system as you slather and spray day after day, hour after hour.

Even when we make an effort to buy the "right" products we are exposed to health-damaging ingredients. Many products don't require FDA approval, and even those that have it (or claim to) are not perfectly safe.

Without suggesting you live in a purified bubble going forward, it's a good idea to be aware of what is on and around our bodies on a daily basis — both tangible and intangible. This includes one of the most toxic (yet invisible) things our bodies sustain...stress. I mention all of these things not in an effort to increase paranoia about the world we live in, but to raise awareness around the fact that it's not just what we put *into* our bodies that affects our health.

TOXINS AND OUR HEALTH

A general toxic overload of our system, or what is known as body burden, is another factor in the relationship between genetics, environment, inflammation, and the gut microbiome.

As we age and our repeated exposures accumulate, the health of our digestive system is compromised (i.e. the gut becomes leaky), leading to decreased resistance to other foreign bodies (like foods to which you have a sensitivity to) and increased inflammation. Such exposures can also affect gene expression — that is, turning on genes that could manifest in disease. Certain genetic variations also exist that significantly lessen the bodies' ability to process or detoxify from toxins and heavy metals.

We've already touched on toxins received directly from our food supply — pesticides and artificial additives — but the effects can be twofold. Chemicals don't just enter your system directly through your mouth, they enter through your skin — the largest organ of your body — and your lungs.

There are now over 3,000 chemicals added to our food supply, and more than 90,000 chemicals used for other purposes in North America. We are inundated with chemical-based products every day — artificial fragrances in room sprays, fabric softeners and cleaning supplies, harmful preservatives in lotions, make-up and hair products...the list goes on, as does the effect from these chemicals as these products are repeatedly slathered on and around our bodies. Heavy metals, one example being mercury, are in our water, potentially in our mouths (via amalgam fillings), and certain kinds of fish. Lead and other compounds are used in many products that surround us.

HEAVY METALS AND ENDOCRINE DISRUPTORS

A heavy metal toxicity can be a leading source of inflammation in many chronic diseases. And certain heavy metals like mercury, lead, and aluminum, can affect our hormones, which puts them in a category known as endocrine disruptors. This simply means they screw up the glands that release hormones into our blood. They affect our male and female sex hormones, playing a large role in fertility issues. They also suppress our thyroid hormones, which not only regulate metabolism, but play a critical role in brain and organ development in infants and young children, and are involved in nearly every physiological process in our bodies.

When the thyroid is sluggish or slow, everything slows down — including the regulation of your immune system. The function of our thyroid also affects our intestinal health, because suppressed thyroid hormones can result in inflammation and a leaky gut...and a leaky gut can lead to inflammation. A vicious circle.

Because of this, hypothyroidism (or a suppressed thyroid) is associated with heart attacks and diabetes, fibromyalgia, irritable bowel syndrome, autoimmune disease, chronic fatigue syndrome, skin conditions (e.g. acne, eczema) and plays an obvious role in various thyroid diseases, including the autoimmune condition Hashimoto's thyroiditis.

In an effort to avoid all of the above issues, we want our thyroid hormones operating on all cylinders, so we need to take note of the following offenders — some fall into the heavy metal category, others do not.

MERCURY

Exposure:

Mercury is a common environmental contaminant. Many of us are exposed to it repeatedly with drinking water, dental amalgams (silver fillings), consuming high-mercury fish (tuna, shark, swordfish, king mackerel, tilefish), certain vaccines and personal care products (e.g. skin-lightening creams, contact lens fluid). It is also found in red tattoo dye.

Effect on Health:

Overexposure to mercury doesn't just affect your thyroid, it can lead to dementia, autism, ADHD and neurological issues. Amalgam fillings* are of particular concern with many international studies confirming adverse health effects. They have been linked to chronic fatigue and many autoimmune diseases, including Hashimoto's thyroiditis and multiple sclerosis.

* The Environmental Protection Agency (EPA) considers mercury fillings that have been removed toxic waste and requires they be disposed as such. Removal should be done only by a biological dentist who will ensure the removed mercury doesn't enter your system during the process. You should also be on a monitored detoxification program with a qualified practitioner to address any mercury that may have been stored in your tissues over time.

LEAD

Exposure:

Lead is another heavy metal that can be found in many things in our environment, including house paint, unfiltered drinking water, and some lipsticks.

Effect on Health:

Besides being an endocrine disruptor, lead has been associated with many other health conditions including: permanent brain damage, lowered IQ, hearing loss, miscarriage, premature birth, hypertension, increased risk of heart disease and strokes, kidney damage, nervous system problems, and lowering your ability to deal with stress.

BISPHENOL A (BPA)

Exposure:

Bisphenol A is a widely-produced chemical primarily used in the production of certain plastics and resins (think plastic bottles, food containers, and disposable coffee cup lids). It is also found in canned foods, and ink from printed receipts.

Effect on Health:

In addition to being an endocrine disruptor, it has been linked to heart disease, obesity and certain cancers (e.g. breast cancer). It is in fact the number one carcinogen in the Environmental Working Group's (EWG) "Dirty Dozen for Cancer Prevention." The National Toxicology Program's Center for the Evaluation of Risks to Human Reproduction (part of the NIH, or National Institutes of Health) has expressed concern for how BPA effects the development of the prostate gland and brain in fetuses, as well as behavioral effects in fetuses, infants and children.

PHTHALATES

Exposure:

Phthalates are found in many personal care and cleaning products, and products made with certain plastics and PVC. They are used in nail polishes to make them chip-resistant and flexible (look for "dibutyl phthalate") and in cosmetics to enhance skin penetration and as moisture enhancers. You will also find them almost anytime you see "fragrance" in the ingredients list (unless it specifically states otherwise). Manufacturers do not have to disclose the ingredients within the fragrance mixture because they are classified as trade secrets by the FDA. They can also be found in our food, namely fast food.

You may see it listed on a label as "DEHP" (diethlyhexyl phthalate) in other products, like plastic shower curtains, rain jackets, and children's toys.

Effect on Health:

As an endocrine disruptor, phthalates are primarily associated with reproductive issues like low sperm count and motility, miscarriage, and infertility in females, as well as hormonal changes in baby boys. However, exposure has also been associated with obesity and insulin resistance in men, and asthma and skin allergies in children.

PFCS

Exposure:

These per- or poly-fluorochemicals are ubiquitous in our environment. We are exposed to them via non-stick cookware, stain repellent, and weather-proof products. They are also used as a coating in fast food wrappers.

Effect on Health:

It has been found that 99% of Americans have these chemicals in their bodies. In addition to being endocrine disruptors, they have been associated with various cancers.

PARABENS

Exposure:

Parabens are pervasive in cosmetics and personal care products, primarily serving as preservatives. They are also sometimes used in packaged foods, beverages, and medications. Look for methyl-, ethyl-, propyl- or butyl-paraben (often at the end of the ingredients list).

Effects on Health:

Beyond the effects of endocrine disruption, they have been linked to skin allergies, skin irritation, and breast cancer.

TRICLOSAN

Exposure:

Triclosan is an artificial antimicrobial chemical that can be found in antibacterial soaps and other cosmetic products like toothpaste and deodorant, dishwasher detergent, and trash bags.

Effect on Health:

While the intent of this synthetic ingredient is to kill germs and prevent the spread of infection, a scientific advisory panel to the FDA determined that antibacterial soaps — including those containing triclosan — were no more effective at killing germs and preventing infection than regular soap. Moreover, the American Medical Association has recommended that triclosan and other antibacterial products not be used for home use due to their association with antibiotic resistance. Over sanitizing can also kill off the *beneficial* bacteria within our microbiome, leading to lowered immunity.

TRIPHENYL PHOSPHATE

Exposure:

Triphenyl phosphate, or TPHP, is the ingredient of concern recently found in many conventional nail polishes. It is listed in the ingredient list of 49% of the nail polishes on the market and also was found in others that made no mention of it. It is also used in fire retardants and plastic manufacturing.

Effect on Health:

Triphenyl phosphate is a suspected endocrine disruptor and currently, research is being done on its role in obesity. In a study performed by Duke University and the EWG, it was found that every study participant that applied a TPHP-containing polish wound up with the chemical in their urine.

KNOWLEDGE IS POWER

Unfortunately, this is only a partial list of ingredients you should be on the look-out for if you want lower the toxic load on your system. New findings and product ingredients are constantly changing. The Roadmap in Chapter 10 will lay out specific actions to take to choose safer products and the Toolkit has a list of other ingredients to avoid and resources to evaluate safety of your current products. You can also find a list of my favorite non-toxic (yet still effective) products on my website at shellymalone.com/inflamed.

CHAPTER 7

HOW STRESS FEEDS DISEASE

Stress. We all have it, we all try to avoid it...and no matter how many foot massages we get, or deep breaths we take, it always comes back to haunt us.

Stress is not easy to manage. There's no magic way to eliminate stress. And there are always other "more important" things to prioritize. Or so we think. I'm hopeful that if you better understand that stress is the gatekeeper of your ability to heal and the specific domino effect it has on your health, you'll make reducing it more of a priority.

Let's look how toxic it can be when we have a constant stressor in our lives — whether that be from personal or financial hardships, an unhealthy relationship or work environment, overtraining your body at the gym, or just spreading yourself too thin in any capacity without adequate rest — and how it all relates to inflammation.

WHAT STRESS REALLY DOES TO YOUR BODY

Acute stress, like acute inflammation, is not necessarily a bad thing. We actually need that instinct. It kicks our "fight or flight" mechanism into gear, alerting us to danger or driving us to meet a deadline. But when stress goes on overload, it becomes chronic — and toxic — in your body.

It all begins in your brain, specifically your hypothalamus. In response to stress, certain hormones are released trickling down to your pituitary gland and then triggering your adrenal glands. The two adrenal glands sitting on top of the kidneys may be small, but they are packing some of the most powerful hormones and neurotransmitters related to energy and stress response. They are chiefly responsible for releasing adrenal steroids, such as cortisol, and the catecholamines (the fight or flight hormones I mentioned, which are officially called epinephrine/adrenalin and norepinephrine). In response to a stressor, the adrenal glands first release adrenaline. Following is the release of cortisol, the "make things happen" hormone that subdues the adrenaline rush and provides you with strength and stamina. This response is meant to be short-lived.

With chronic, prolonged stress, cortisol and adrenaline are pumped too high, too frequently. These constant levels not only keep us overly riled up emotionally, they have significant physical impacts including suppressing our immune system and increasing the permeability of our gut. Multiple studies have shown that stress changes gene expression in immune cells making them more inflammatory. And at a certain point, your adrenal glands won't be able to keep up with the demand for cortisol, which can lead to lethargy, mood and cognitive issues, digestive conditions, food sensitivities, low sex drive, food cravings, and many other undesirable symptoms. You may have heard of this condition referred to as adrenal fatigue; however, the more accurate is HPA (hypothalamus, pituitary, adrenal) -axis dysfunction. Keep in mind that stress from physical illness and food sensitivities previously discussed are also considered stressors and follow a similar physiological path to destruction.

With this cascade of destruction, you cannot dismiss the important role decreasing your stress plays in your body's ability to heal. Add in nutrient deficiencies from not consuming enough high-nutrient, unprocessed foods (like fresh vegetables), low quality animal protein from animals not raised on amino acid and anti-inflammatory omega-3 rich grass, too much sugar or caffeine, or food additives that are inhibiting your brain chemistry to adapt to stress — and you've created a perfect storm of devastation to your overall health.

CHAPTER 7

SLEEP AND REST: CRITICAL, BUT OFTEN IGNORED

Sleep is a major factor in your stress level and response to stress.

In general, life can be exhausting. And anyone suffering from a chronic, inflammatory condition is likely all too familiar with fatigue. While eliminating sources of inflammation as best you can through your diet, environment, and the products you use is integral, you can't overlook the basic practice of getting enough rest. A multitude of studies show that lack of sleep — even mild or short-term deprivation — can increase inflammation and contribute to chronic disease, with those that consistently get less than seven hours of sleep per day most at risk. Yet, we often dismiss its importance and the factors that contribute to its loss.

Research has also shown that lack of sleep has effects on your hormones and brain function causing you to crave high sugar and junk foods, which ultimately lead to an increase in inflammatory insulin production.

Rest also pertains to your workout routine. If you have a hard time recovering from a workout, if you have to drag yourself to do the workout itself, or if you're gaining weight despite an increase in exercise, these are all signs you're overdoing it. Sometimes you need to stop working so hard against yourself, so your body can start working for you.

OBSTACLES TO SLEEP

EXCESS CAFFEINE

It's going to be pretty hard to get the rest you need if you're downing three triple lattes a day.

While the benefits of coffee have been shown in studies, and highly touted in the media, those benefits could be due to the high antioxidant content, which could easily be attained from eating whole foods, in particular fruits and vegetables. And while coffee may be fine for some, if you have inflammation, stress, or fatigue, coffee will do you more harm than good.

When you consume coffee, sodas, or energy drinks with a high caffeine content, your stress hormones (catecholamines) are increased, which can cause spikes in blood sugar. This results in corresponding spikes of insulin which then increases inflammation. Ultimately, you feel even more drained because you are taxing your adrenal glands, which play a vital role in your energy and stress response.

ARTIFICIAL LIGHT

One often overlooked cause of poor sleep is exposure to artificial light, or blue light from computer screens and mobile devices. A 2014 study revealed that we are spending an average of 7.4 hours in front of a screen every day in the U.S.: 2.5 hours spent watching television, 1.7 in front of a computer, 2.5 hours on a smart phone and 43 minutes on a tablet. The effect of this — besides the cognitive deficits beyond the scope of this book — is a significant decrease in our levels of melatonin, the hormone made in the brain that controls our sleep and wake cycles.

CHAPTER 8:

HOW YOUR PAST MEDICAL HISTORY CAN CONTRIBUTE TO POOR HEALTH

Stemming from our current health system's focus on treatment rather than prevention, some of our well-meaning conventional treatments have actually been detrimental to our chronic health conditions. This is not to say that they weren't or aren't necessary to address acute issues, but it is important to recognize the long-term effects they have on our nutrient status and gut health, and their role in inflammation. In many cases we can make changes that allow us to focus on the root cause of the issue, move forward, and most importantly, heal.

Below are common culprits from the past that affect our present health.

C-SECTION BIRTH

When a baby passes through the birth canal during a normal vaginal birth, s/he swallows fluid from the birth canal on the way down and in doing so "inoculates" their gut with mom's gut flora, including the beneficial, or commensal bacteria (like lactobacillus).

If the baby is born via C-section, s/he skips this critical step and can instead inherit the pathogenic make-up of the hospital flora environment. In addition, the antibiotics mom receives during and after the procedure are passed on to baby, further altering the gut flora (AKA gut microbiome)

The immune system goes through major development during infancy and the microbiome plays a huge role in this. With C-section rates rapidly increasing — 33% of all births in the U.S. as of 2013 — concurrent with an epidemic of autoimmune disease (e.g. type I diabetes, Crohn's disease, multiple sclerosis) and allergic disease such as asthma, allergic rhinitis, and atopic dermatitis, it is hypothesized that there is a correlation.

LACK OF BREASTMILK

Before the firestorm starts, know this: this is NOT about mom-shaming. Just knowledge. Simply putting pieces together. I have worked in the NICU and know the physiological issues that can prevent exclusive breastfeeding — whether it's health issues with mom or baby. And I am well aware of obstacles faced by all Moms in their pursuit to nourish their infants with breastmilk, including inadequate maternity leave benefits, lack of support and misinformation from practitioners, societal pressures and sub-par public facilities.

Breast milk, or human milk, is a vehicle for critical protective bacteria as well as other important immunological properties like lysozyme, secretory IgA, and leukocytes. Breastmilk will even change in its make-up of antibodies to address the specific illness in the child. They don't call it "liquid gold" for nothing. It is essential — especially during the first six months — because during this time an infants' tight junctions aren't yet closed. In essence, the babies gut is born leaky. It is the early milk — the colostrum

— and then the continuation of breast milk that aids in sealing these up. This is why the nutrition an infant receives is critical to setting the scene for their microbiome. If an infant is instead receiving formula (made with cow's milk protein), they are not only *not* sealing up the tight junctions for a healthy gut, they are also at the mercy of the inflammatory casein in cow's milk. There is a dose-response effect with breastmilk (the more received, the better the outcomes), but in general, being breastfed is associated with a reduced risk of: ear infections, GI infections, respiratory tract infections, dermatitis, childhood asthma, childhood leukemia, type 1 diabetes, obesity, and sudden infant death syndrome (SIDS). It is also hypothesized that lack of breastmilk plays a role in autoimmune disease and overall immunity.

EXCESS ANTI-INFLAMMATORIES AND PAIN RELIEVERS

A common approach, especially with exclusive exposure to conventional medicine ideals, is that management of inflammation is through quick-fix anti-inflammatory medications like NSAIDS (Non-Steroidal Anti-Inflammatory Drugs). These include prescription NSAIDS and over-the-counter ibuprofen and naproxen. It is well supported in the research that this particular class of pain relievers is very damaging to your digestive system and can increase the permeability of your gut. Prescription corticosteroids can also have the same effect. Ironically (and unfortunately), these are commonly prescribed for autoimmune and other inflammatory conditions and exacerbates a root cause — a leaky gut.

Both fish oil and curcumin have been found to be as effective for treating pain as NSAIDs in several studies. One of the most effective, natural anti-inflammatories is the bright-yellow culinary spice turmeric (active component: curcumin). Turmeric is the main spice in curry and the reason mustard is yellow. It has more than two dozen anti-inflammatory compounds and its benefits have been widely studied. Turmeric has been shown to outperform many pharmaceuticals in its effective fight against several chronic, debilitating diseases with virtually no side effects, including: arthritis (including rheumatoid arthritis), fibromyalgia, Alzheimer's disease, certain cancers, depression, inflammatory skin conditions, gallbladder and liver disorders, bronchitis, heartburn, and more.

OVERUSE OF ANTIBIOTICS

Antibiotics are another common first defense for chronic issues related to infections. While these absolutely have their place, the underlying cause of chronic infections are not typically addressed. So while antibiotics treat many things thought to be associated with inflammation, they disrupt the microbiome because they do a clean sweep, taking the good bacteria with the bad. Just one course has been found to permanently alter your gut flora. Five days on a broad spectrum antibiotic removes one-third of beneficial bacteria that you won't get back. So, antibiotics, like NSAIDS, perpetuate the root cause of the issue—making your gut even leakier, leading toxins and foods you don't tolerate right into your system, and then inappropriately triggering an inflammatory, or immune response. And if you're also eating conventional animal products, you are already consuming a large amount of these microbiome-disrupting medications through your diet.

CHRONIC USE OF PROTON-PUMP INHIBITORS (ANTACIDS)

These commonly taken medications work by inhibiting gastric acid production. This can be quite effective for reflux and heartburn (aka GERD) in the short-term. However, because they lead to many vitamin & mineral deficiencies and decrease the acidity in the stomach that acts as a protectant to pathogenic bacteria, long-term use has been linked to increased osteoporosis and hip fractures, dementia, decreased resistance to infections with a specific increase in *Clostridium difficile* and *H. Pylori* infections (harmful, pathogenic bacteria), irritable bowel syndrome and small intestinal bacterial overgrowth (SIBO). There are also some reports that long-term use could be associated with esophageal and stomach cancers.

Reflux can often be addressed with diet and lifestyle factors:

- Avoiding spicy foods, caffeine and fried foods, or citrus for some people
- Identifying and eliminating food sensitivities (especially gluten and dairy, possibly FODMAPs)
- Not eating right before bed
- Reducing stress
- Losing weight, if needed

A variety of nutritional supplements can also be effective depending on the individual, including probiotics, magnesium, hydrochloric acid, bitter herbs, apple cider vinegar or digestive enzymes.

Common Drugs and Associated Nutrient Deficiencies

Anti-Inflammatories (cortico-steroids and NSAIDs)	Calcium, Vitamin D, Magnesium, Zinc, Vitamin C, Vitamin B12, Folic Acid, Selenium, Iron, Potassium
Antibiotics	B Vitamins, Vitamin K, Calcium, Magnesium, Iron, Zinc
Antacids	Vitamin B12, Folic Acid, Calcium, Iron, Zinc
Cardiovascular Drugs	Coenzyme Q10, Vitamin B1, Vitamin B6, Zinc
Female Hormones (contraceptives, hormone replacement/estrogen)	Vitamin B2, B3, B6, B12, Folic Acid, Vitamin C, Magnesium, Selenium, Zinc
Anti-Depressants	Coenzyme Q10, Vitamin B2

LONG-TERM OR EXCESSIVE ALCOHOL USE

In a Harvard study, it was found that alcohol kills an average of 100,000 people per year (excluding deaths from alcohol-related car accidents and crimes).

Chronic alcohol use impairs the function of your gut and liver (your primary detoxifying organ) as well as disrupts multiple organ interactions which leads to persistent, systemic inflammation. Alcohol can also increase estrogen levels in women. It has also been shown that women who have three alcoholic drinks per week have a 15%

higher risk of breast cancer, with the risk going up an additional 10% for each additional drink consumed per day. Not to mention alcohol is an extremely refined carbohydrate which creates blood sugar imbalances and inflammatory insulin spikes when consumed.

CIGARETTE SMOKING

Cigarette smoking kills nearly 500,000 people each year and takes 13–15 years off of an adult life. While it is commonly known that smoking causes lung cancer, chronic lung disease, cardiovascular disease and oral disease, it is important to realize that cigarette smoke can cause cancer almost anywhere in the body. It is made up of thousands of chemicals that alter gene expression (waking up disease-prone genes), and promotes chronic inflammation while also suppressing your immune response to pathogens. It is also thought to promote certain autoimmune diseases, including RA.

Other relevant medical history that can contribute to a disrupted microbiome and chronic inflammation include:

- hidden or chronic infections (yeast, viruses, bacteria or parasites)
- mercury amalgams (silver fillings) — See Chapter 7
- radiation or chemotherapy

The nature of the conditions you may be suffering from — and the treatment of them — can vary greatly. Your genetics and biochemistry are also very individual as is your current nutrient status. You should always work with a qualified health practitioner to customize a treatment plan, especially if your goal is to transition away from conventional medication. The Toolkit includes links to help you find a progressive practitioner (e.g. integrative, functional, holistic physician, naturopathic doctor (ND), or other qualified clinician) that will focus treatment on the root cause of your issues.

FOCUS ON WHAT YOU CAN CONTROL

Remember: knowledge is power.

While a lot of this may be hard to hear, it's critical for you to bravely dive into the information so you can understand the interplay between your gut, the environment, and your genes, and how it all combines to create a template for your overall health and well-being. We can't live in the past. All we can do is recognize, and learn from our experiences.

PART THREE
EXTINGUISH

CHAPTER 9:

GETTING STARTED: LIGHTING THE PATH FOR LIFESTYLE CHANGE

Now that you've read about how our lifestyles interconnect with our overall well-being, you have a big picture and some framework within which to start putting some real change into effect — modifications that will, step by step, come together to create a new way of living. You've replaced ineffective sound bites with solid information about how you feel and why. Appreciate the powerful knowledge you now have and understand that going forward, it's up to you to implement the changes you need in your life, in order to realize your optimal good health.

You know you best — what your life looks like on a daily, weekly, and monthly basis. And you know all too well just how you've been feeling and how ready you are (or aren't) to make changes in your life.

You're in prime position to take action. And now you might be thinking, "Okay, I've got all the information...what in the HELL am I supposed to do with it?!"

I will provide you a roadmap to follow — a detailed change management system.

But, I'm not talking about implementing swaps for a week or two to "cleanse" or "reset" your system. I'm talking about lifelong, consistent change.

CHANGE MANAGEMENT

Making change sustainable is not easy. To do it successfully — and here I equate success with the least amount of pain and the best outcomes — requires adequate planning and addressing many factors, some of which may not be obvious.

According to the managing complex change model by Ambrose (1987), there are five critical elements required for a big change to be successful: vision, skills, incentive, resources, and an action plan. In order to effect a positive change instead of a negative one, you need all five elements to be in place. Without any one of them, you will end up with a less than optimal outcome.

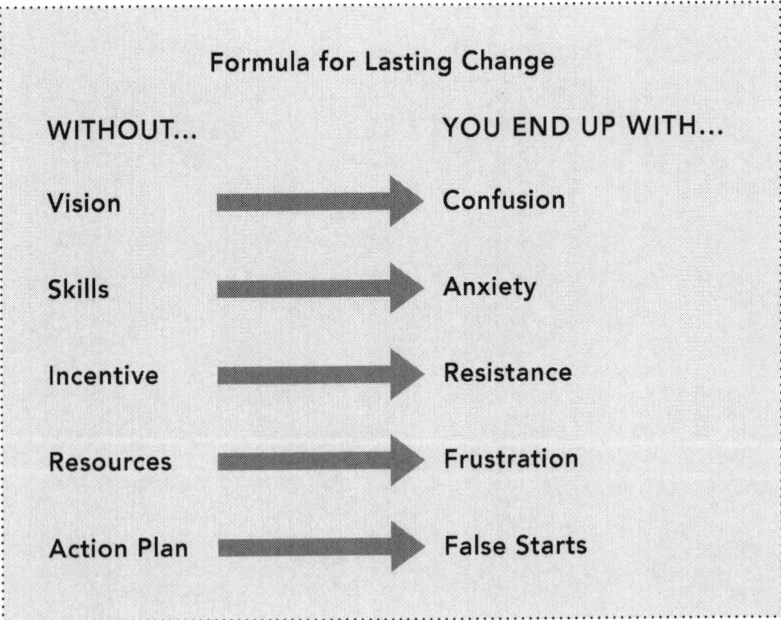

Let's apply each of these elements to our goal: to alter your diet and lifestyle in order to reduce inflammation.

VISION

After reading the first two parts of this book, can you visualize how your diet and lifestyle contribute to inflammation and chronic disease from a big picture standpoint? Do you understand how and why implementing progressive practices consistently will deliver better health outcomes?

Without a bigger vision, or context, we end up with confusion and random actions based on a momentary inspiration from something we read or hear. It's important to acknowledge that the media hype that's tossed at us is just bits and pieces of whatever will raise viewership—with no context. And it's most definitely not tailored to our lives, so while it sounds convincing, it's not always relevant. For example, there is no virtue in buying gluten-free donuts, just because we heard a news story about it. Coconut oil is a great ingredient but remember why you need to use it before you add it into your flour-laden sugar cookie recipe.

SKILLS

Do you know now what specific diet and lifestyle factors you need to implement to reduce inflammation? Do you know what to look for on a label, whether on food, cosmetic, or household product packaging? How to plan meals, then cook and eat a balanced diet?

Your answers are of value, because being able to see that your diet and lifestyle can make you sick is only one part. It needs to be combined with knowledge. Without knowing what to do about how you feel, you can end up feeling anxious, overwhelmed, and frozen. The first two sections of the book got you halfway there. We're going to finish it off in our upcoming Roadmap and Toolkit.

INCENTIVE

I like to call this your "Why." Why are you reading this book? Why would you inconvenience yourself by implementing these changes? Resist giving yourself generic answers like "It's healthy" or "It's good for me" or "My mom/wife/husband/friend wants me to do this." Spend some time and go deeper.

Keep asking "Why" after every answer you give to yourself, peeling the layers back until you reveal what is really at the core of your desire to learn and change. Think about your life without the pain, fatigue, skin issues, depression, living at the doctor's office, or whatever your condition might be bringing to you. How would your life be different if those were eliminated?

RESOURCES

So now you see the big picture. You know why you need to improve your diet or lifestyle, and you understand exactly what you need to do, but let's talk about the required resources. Resources could range from money ("Grass-fed beef isn't in my budget"), to checklists and reminders ("Which fruits and vegetables should I buy organic?"), to shortcuts for shopping for and preparing meals due to physical impairments — pain or otherwise.

Knowing what to do, but not being able to do it, leads to frustration. In the Toolkit, I provide informational cheat sheets, and ideas on eating healthy on a budget, as well as time-saving tips. Part of building your personal roadmap might be working on your spending priorities (and returning to your *Why* in the process).

ACTION PLAN

You could have all the knowledge, resources and incentive in the world, but if you don't have a plan that sets you on a clear path towards accomplishing your goals, your fresh start could turn into a false start at the first roadblock.

I made this mistake myself after first being diagnosed and learning the role of diet in inflammation. I threw myself into drastic changes without having a specific action plan. I eliminated all common food sensitivities, drastically reduced sugar, and started eating organic/non-GMO. But, while my pain and fatigue were diminishing quickly, my diet was out of balance. I was hungry and miserable because I hadn't planned out substitutions. The only thing that saved me from a nosedive right after take-off was the fact that I knew I needed this change to survive.

Part of your action plan is readying answers to questions that will come up along the way, tempting you to go back to your old, unhealthy patterns. In order to effect lifelong change, you'll need to adopt the long view — and be ready to stay the course — as you prepare your roadmap to success.

SETTING GOALS YOU WILL ACHIEVE

Achievement feels good. When we achieve a goal — no matter how small it is — our brain releases the happy hormone dopamine which provides us with greater concentration and motivates us to continue the same activity that caused the initial release of the hormone. This is why it feels so good to check a box off of your to-do list. Conversely, every time you fail to achieve a goal, the release of dopamine slows, killing your motivation. So it makes sense to break your goals down into small, individual steps and collect some little wins first.

The Roadmap is broken into 25 goals with small, very specific ideas for action to help you reach each one. Let the momentum (and the dopamine release) from achieving the small goals push you towards bigger goals that you might have been previously resistant to working towards. Eventually, little wins lead to big wins. And the biggest win — vibrant and healthy living — is what all of this is about.

If you implemented one goal every two weeks, by this time next year you could be feeling like a new person altogether. Chances are, you'll start feeling better long before that though…and you're always able to put yourself on a fast track if you're ready for a more aggressive change strategy.

It's time to take your newfound knowledge and your *Why* to the starting line. Where will you begin this journey of change? Maybe you are already a great cook, incorporating vegetables and avoiding most gluten or dairy. Or maybe (like me) you are really good at eliminating inflammatory items from your life and diet, but aren't as good at adding in beneficial, inflammation-fighting foods and practices or addressing the stress in your life.

Be honest with yourself about where your starting point is, so you can start by picking the low hanging fruit, getting some easy wins and building momentum towards the bigger ones. If you fall off the wagon, come back to this tool. Reassess and jump back on where it feels most appropriate.

My hope is that you use this Roadmap for years to come, to help maintain a lifestyle that allows you to thrive.

CHAPTER 10:

ANTI-INFLAMMATORY ROADMAP: 25 STEPS TO VIBRANT HEALTH

Think of this as your step-by-step guide to cleaning up your diet, reducing inflammation, and feeling a lot better. While we will revisit the concepts we covered in Part Two, the focus here is on action. This is where you apply the information in order to make changes in your daily life.

Read through all 25 goals and then decide for yourself where you'd like to start. The goals are presented in an order that addresses a few easy-to-implement, foundational steps to start and then built upon from there. You can combine a couple, or just pick one and implement it for two weeks, then move on to your next goal. This does not dictate the absolute path for any one individual. Where you are now — what your diet and lifestyle practices look like and how ready you are to change — should be your guide. For most of the steps, you'll find corresponding guides or other helpful information in the Toolkit that you can refer to along the way as well. The guides from the Toolkit and more can also be downloaded at shellymalone.com/inflamed.

Keep in mind, some goals are going to have a much bigger impact than others. For example, changing your salt is not going to have the immediate impact on inflammation that say, eliminating foods you are sensitive to will. Also note that some of these items can be treated with more of an 80/20 approach. Working on decreasing pesticides and other toxins as much as possible, whenever possible will help lower your body burden. And others, like removing gluten and conventional dairy and any other known sensitivities will need to be approached with a more absolute stance on elimination for the long term.

But don't lose the forest for the trees — each individual step plays a key role in reducing the inflammatory impacts on your entire system. You will be lowering the amounts of toxins going in, on and around your body day after day. You'll ensure the highest nutritional content of the foods you're consuming. You will increase antioxidants and reduce the stress (in all forms) that hampers your immunity.

GOAL 1:
CLEAN UP YOUR WATER (AND DRINK ENOUGH OF IT)

WHY

Water should be your primary source for hydration, so it makes sense to ensure it is from a good source.

- Tap water can contain arsenic, aluminum, excess chlorine and fluoride, other heavy metals and endocrine disruptors, even traces of discarded medications.
- Plastic water bottles can contain another endocrine disruptor and carcinogen, BPA.
- Adequate water intake assists with excreting excess toxins in your system.

IDEAS FOR ACTION

- [ ] Buy a home water filter or buy outside filtered water (reverse osmosis systems with a carbon filter are currently viewed as the most effective method).
- [ ] Stop purchasing and drinking from BPA-containing plastic water bottles, opting for glass, stainless steel or BPA-free bottles/containers.
- [ ] Drink 6–8 glasses of water per day to assist with excretion of toxins (or enough for your pee to run clear).

FOR MORE GUIDANCE

Environmental Working Group's (EWG) "Water Filter Buying Guide"

GOAL 2:
CLEAN UP YOUR SALT

WHY

When you choose the better, unrefined source, salt is no longer the enemy to run from, it is actually a healthful, essential part of your diet.

- Table salt is over-processed, containing bleaching and anti-caking chemicals and aluminum.
- Unlike table salt, sea salt retains many vital minerals, like magnesium and potassium, which balance the level of sodium.

IDEAS FOR ACTION

- [ ] Swap conventional table (even Kosher) salt for Celtic or Himalayan sea salt.
- [ ] Consider an iodine-fortified brand of sea salt, if supplementation has been recommended for a thyroid condition.

FOR MORE GUIDANCE

Toolkit: "Pantry Staples to Stock"

GOAL 3:
EAT ORGANIC AND NON-GMO WHENEVER POSSIBLE

WHY

Organic produce has been shown to have higher levels of inflammation-fighting antioxidants than non-organic produce (up to three times the levels if it is seasonal) and will significantly limit your consumption of pesticides and GMOs which can cause systemic damage to your body.

- An organic label will ensure that the product doesn't contain synthetic solvents if "artificial" or "natural flavors" are listed in the ingredient list.
- Avoiding foods made from genetically-modified organisms (GMOs) will also reduce exposure to gut-damaging Bt-toxins.

IDEAS FOR ACTION

- ☐ Buy organic produce based on the EWG Shopping Guides for "Clean 15/Dirty Dozen" and "Shoppers Guide to Avoiding GMOs".
- ☐ Join a community supporting agricultural (CSA) program to receive local, organic produce.
- ☐ Buy produce from your local Farmer's Market.
- ☐ Plant your own produce and herbs.
- ☐ Avoid all corn and soy, unless it specifically states non-GMO.

- [ ] Consume quality animal protein (see Goal 4).

- [ ] Switch to organic coffee.

FOR MORE GUIDANCE

Toolkit: “Guide to Organic” and “Guide to GMOs”

GOAL 4:
CHOOSE QUALITY ANIMAL PROTEIN

WHY

Avoiding pesticides and GMOs includes avoiding the animal products that receive them in their feed.

- If animals aren't raised in pasture, they don't have room to roam or grass to eat to increase their levels of anti-inflammatory omega-3 fats and important fat-soluble vitamins A & D.
- Farmed fish will have higher levels of carcinogens and other contaminants.
- Nitrates from processed meats are a probable carcinogen.

IDEAS FOR ACTION

- [ ] Choose beef, bison, chicken, eggs, and dairy that are organic and grass-fed (ideally 100% grass-fed to be sure the animals aren't also fed grains), or pastured.
- [ ] Choose wild seafood and avoid fish with high mercury levels.
- [ ] Choose whole meats over processed whenever possible. If purchasing processed meats, look for labels calling out "nitrate-free," "no nitrates," or "uncured."
- [ ] If you don't have access to these foods at your local stores or Farmer's Market, use a delivery service.
- [ ] If budget is an issue, prioritize the product(s) you eat most often (and remember, animal protein should only make up about 25% of each meal).

FOR MORE GUIDANCE

Toolkit: "Product Labels"; shellymalone.com/inflamed: "Whole Food Delivery"; "EWG's Consumer Guide to Seafood"

GOAL 5:
EAT MORE (GOOD) FATS

WHY

Eating enough of the right kind of fat is an essential part of an anti-inflammatory diet:

- It regulates blood sugar (balancing inflammatory insulin).
- It promotes tissue healing (including gut tissue) and immune function.
- It aids in making vitamin D (a common deficiency in chronic disease).

IDEAS FOR ACTION

- [ ] Make sure you get at least a serving of fat at each meal.
- [ ] Use the following liquid oils: organic, cold-pressed extra virgin olive, macadamia, flax, and avocado oils.
- [ ] Use the following solid fats: coconut oil, organic/grass-fed ghee or butter (only if you can tolerate casein), non-hydrogenated palm oil, and pastured sources of animal fats.
- [ ] Avoid corn, soy, and other vegetable oils and partially-hydrogenated fats and margarine.
- [ ] Take a daily omega-3 supplement (caution if on blood thinning or anti-hypertensive medication).
- [ ] Consume a serving of wild-caught salmon or other wild caught, low-mercury fish 2 times per week.

- [ ] Purchase grass-fed or pastured beef, eggs, bison.
- [ ] Include walnuts, chia and flax seeds (ideally soaked in filtered water overnight) in a daily smoothie.
- [ ] Stop purchasing and consuming low-fat products.

FOR MORE GUIDANCE

Toolkit: "Pantry Staples to Stock," "Which Fats When"

GOAL 6:
LIMIT ALL SUGAR AND AVOID PROCESSED SUGAR

WHY

Refined sugar is one of the most damaging ingredients you can consume and it has effects on your entire system.

- Consuming sugar increases inflammatory insulin levels.
- Sugar feeds the pathogenic (bad) bacteria in your gut microbiome, leading to dysbiosis and a leaky gut.
- 95% of sugar beet crops (where much of your table sugar comes from unless specifically stated as "pure cane sugar" or coming from alternative sources) are genetically modified.

Ideally, all forms of sugar should be reduced as much as possible, but natural forms are safer and can offer nutritional benefits like minerals and antioxidants.

IDEAS FOR ACTION

- [ ] Cut down on obvious sugary treats — reduce portions and frequency and focus on conscious eating (savoring every bite).
- [ ] Replace conventional sweets with less sugary options like dark chocolate (at least 70% cacao) or fresh berries.
- [ ] Avoid sugary sodas or damaging artificial sweeteners by swapping plain filtered water, club soda or mineral water for the fountain machine.

- [ ] Stop eating all processed sugar (especially high fructose corn syrup) swapping for natural sweeteners like raw honey, coconut or palm sugar, organic maple syrup, molasses, stevia, or Lakanto sugar.

- [ ] In recipes, swap sugar options above.

- [ ] Choose whole fruits over juices or dried fruits.

- [ ] Choose natural condiments and salad dressings.

- [ ] Slowly reduce all sweeteners, even the natural forms, in everything you eat and drink.

FOR MORE GUIDANCE

Toolkit: "Pantry Staples to Stock," "Lesser Evils"

GOAL 7:
REBALANCE YOUR CARBS AND ANIMAL PROTEIN

WHY

Previous guidelines to eat a high carbohydrate diet result in increases of inflammatory insulin and can be damaging to your gut lining.

Animal protein has a wealth of key nutrients and when eaten in the appropriate amounts, can decrease inflammation.

IDEAS FOR ACTION

- ☐ Make grains/starches no more than 25% of each meal:
  - ☐ Swap traditional gluten-containing grains for root vegetables, like sweet potato or yucca.
  - ☐ Use a spiralizer to replace grains with zucchini or other vegetables.
  - ☐ Try spaghetti squash as a pasta replacement.
  - ☐ Try cauliflower rice or cauliflower mashed "potatoes."
  - ☐ Enjoy open-faced sandwiches.
  - ☐ Use leafy greens for sandwich wraps
- ☐ Ideally, make all grains gluten-free and have them soaked or sprouted whenever possible.
- ☐ When you consume animal protein, aim for it to make-up about 25% of each meal.

FOR MORE GUIDANCE

Toolkit: "Recipe Resources" and "Easy Dishes"; shellymalone.com/inflamed: "Favorite Products"

GOAL 8:
EAT MORE VEGETABLES (ESPECIALLY DARK GREEN VEGETABLES)

WHY

These nutritional powerhouses provide many essential vitamins and minerals, including vitamin E (a potent inflammation-fighter), B vitamins, disease-fighting phytonutrients, calcium and fiber.

IDEAS FOR ACTION

- ☐ Aim for each meal to be 50% vegetables and fruit (mostly vegetables) and try to get 5–7 servings per day, choosing from a variety of colors.
- ☐ Spend about 30 minutes 1–2 times per week baking or roasting vegetables in olive oil or coconut oil for use throughout the week — with eggs in the morning, a side for lunch or dinner, in a salad, etc.
- ☐ Swap a cold-pressed green juice or green smoothie for a coffee in the morning or afternoon 3–7 times per week. (If you gag on the taste, suck it down with a straw.)
- ☐ Add Tuscan or Lacinato kale to a morning fruit smoothie (you can barely taste it).
- ☐ Learn a new vegetable recipe each week.
- ☐ Find a green food supplement you can add to water or non-dairy milk.
- ☐ Sign-up for a weekly CSA produce delivery and commit to using everything in the box.

FOR MORE GUIDANCE

Toolkit: "Recipe Resources"; shellymalone.com/inflamed: "Favorite Products"

GOAL 9:
LIMIT TOXINS FROM FOOD

WHY

Beyond pesticides and GMOs, our food — especially processed food and the packaging its served in — can be a huge source of additives and chemicals. These can have varying effects on our health, from ADHD to cancer, and add to your bodies overall toxic load.

IDEAS FOR ACTION

- [ ] Avoid any packaged food with artificial sweeteners, artificial colors or flavors, MSG, nitrates, BHT/BHA, or high fructose corn syrup on the label.
- [ ] Avoid canned foods unless it specifically states it is BPA-free, opting for products in glass or tetra-paks.
- [ ] Avoid microwave popcorn.
- [ ] Limit consumption of rice products to avoid arsenic.
- [ ] Make your own bread or purchase from a bakery you trust to avoid potassium bromate.
- [ ] Swap table salt for sea salt.
- [ ] Use aluminum-free baking powder.
- [ ] Cook meats at lower temperatures (braising, baking, etc.) and marinate your meat in a liquid with plenty of herbs and spices (particularly rosemary) before barbecuing to reduce carcinogenic amine formation.

- [ ] Avoid high-mercury fish (king mackerel, shark, swordfish, tile fish, orange roughy, marlin).

- [ ] Work up a sweat multiple times a week with exercise and take Epsom salt baths to help detoxify from toxins.

FOR MORE GUIDANCE

Toolkit: "Pantry Staples to Stock," "Product Labels"; shellymalone.com/inflamed: "Favorite Products"

GOAL 10:
SAY GOOD-BYE TO GLUTEN

WHY

Gluten is a very common food sensitivity and source for inflammation that is linked to over 50 disease states.

- When consumed, it releases a protein that unzips the tight junctions of your intestines which can lead to a leaky gut in those predisposed.

- When there is a sensitivity, gluten must be eliminated completely. The smallest amount could illicit inflammation and take weeks to months to repair the intestinal tissue damage.

IDEAS FOR ACTION

Get Prepared:

- ☐ Use the Toolkit to find out which products have gluten in them and find replacements, focusing on whole foods that are naturally gluten-free: whole vegetables, fruits, nuts, seeds, beans, starches like sweet potatoes, ancient grains, and rice.

- ☐ Search for whole, gluten-free recipes that sound good.

- ☐ Shop for your new gluten-free substitutes and plan meals at least 3 days ahead.

- ☐ Research gluten-free items at restaurants near you.

- ☐ After steps 1–4 are completed, take gluten completely out of your diet (not a crumb!) for at least two weeks (ideally four to six).

- [ ] Take a DPPIV digestive enzyme whenever you eat out in case of inadvertent gluten contamination.

- [ ] Keep track of your symptoms each day. If symptoms resolve, it is best to not reintroduce gluten.

If symptoms do not resolve, keep in mind that you may also have a sensitivity to dairy/casein or another food in addition to gluten that is not allowing you to see the full benefit. Ideally, take gluten, dairy/casein and soy out of your diet at the same time.

FOR MORE GUIDANCE

Toolkit: "Navigating Gluten," "Recipe Resources," "Pantry Staples to Stock," "Easy Dishes," "On-The-Go Snacks"; shellymalone.com/inflamed: "Favorite Products," "Elimination Diet Template"

GOAL 11:
REMOVE PASTEURIZED COW'S MILK

WHY

Like gluten, casein from cow's milk is another very common food sensitivity. And the way conventional cow's milk is processed, and the type of casein today's cow produces, combine to make it very pro-inflammatory and harmful to your microbiome.

IDEAS FOR ACTION

Get Prepared:

- ☐ Use the Toolkit to find out which products have casein in them and find replacements.
- ☐ Search for whole, dairy-free recipes that sound appealing.
- ☐ Shop for your new dairy-free substitutes (nut, hemp or rice milk-based products) and plan meals at least 3 days ahead.
- ☐ Research dairy-free items at restaurants near you.
- ☐ After steps 1–4 are completed, take all dairy/casein completely out of your diet for at least 2 weeks (ideally 4).
- ☐ Keep track of your symptoms each day.
- ☐ If symptoms resolve, you can try to introduce a small serving once per day of a more tolerated casein product, like organic, raw goat or sheep's milk or grass-fed butter, and see if you have any type of reaction.
- ☐ If no symptoms or reaction occur with raw goat or sheep's milk, you can try a small serving per day of raw, grass-fed cow's milk.

If your symptoms don't resolve, keep in mind that you could also have a sensitivity to gluten or another food that is not allowing you to see the full benefit from removing casein.

FOR MORE GUIDANCE

Toolkit: "Navigating Dairy," "Recipe Resources," "Pantry Staples to Stock," "Easy Dishes," "On-The-Go Snacks"; shellymalone.com/inflamed: "Favorite Products," "Elimination Diet Template"; shellymalone.com/how-and-why-i-broke-up-with-dairy

GOAL 12:
LOOK FOR OTHER FOOD SENSITIVITIES

WHY

While gluten and dairy are often the biggest culprits, food sensitivities can be from many different foods and food categories and are a big cause of inflammation.

Ideas for Action:

- ☐ Make an appointment with an integrative or functional dietitian or other practitioner familiar with assessing food sensitivities and implementing elimination diets so that you can maintain a healthful, balanced diet while looking for foods to which you are sensitive.

- ☐ If you are unable to see a practitioner, use the "Elimination Diet Guide" and other guides listed below to implement yourself. I recommend starting this after you have tried eliminating gluten, dairy and soy simultaneously for 2–6 weeks.

FOR MORE GUIDANCE

Toolkit: "Pantry Staples to Stock," "Recipe Resources," "Easy Dishes," "On-The-Go Snacks"; shellymalone.com/inflamed: "Favorite Products," "Elimination Diet Template"

GOAL 13:
BUILD A HEALTHY MICROBIOME

WHY

Adding to your beneficial (commensal) bacteria and helping to heal a leaky gut can improve your ability to absorb nutrients, prevent toxins and pathogens from entering the bloodstream and eliminate some food sensitivities — all reducing inflammation.

IDEAS FOR ACTION

- [ ] Take 1 multi-strain probiotic/day (10–25 billion CFU's) that includes lactobacillus and bifidobacterium. If you have yeast (candida) it should only contain the strain, *Saccharomyces boulardi.*

- [ ] Incorporate foods into your diet that act as prebiotics (feed beneficial bacteria): garlic, leeks, onion, dandelion greens, Jerusalem artichoke, asparagus, yams or sweet potatoes.

- [ ] Integrate a serving of fermented vegetables (e.g. kimchi, sauerkraut) into your meals at least a few times per week – either homemade or purchased at your Farmer's Market or natural grocery store.

- [ ] Swap soda and juice for kombucha (fermented tea).

- [ ] Consume organic, grass-fed meat or bone broth (sip alone or use for soups).

- [ ] Swap regular hot sauce for a fermented version.

- [ ] Stop using antimicrobial products for non-acute issues (especially those that contain triclosan).

- [ ] Consider switching to oil-based soaps, like castile.
- [ ] Soak your (gluten-free) grains or seeds overnight before eating.
- [ ] Consider taking a digestive enzyme before meals or drinking lemon water after meals to aid in digestion.

FOR MORE GUIDANCE

Toolkit: "Recipe Resources"; shellymalone.com/inflamed: "Favorite Products"

Important note: If you have been diagnosed with SIBO or an intolerance to histamines or FODMAPS — or suspect you may have any of these conditions — do not start probiotics, fermented foods, bone broths or start incorporating prebiotic foods regularly without first consulting with a qualified health practitioner familiar with digestive health.

GOAL 14:
CHANGE OUT YOUR PERSONAL CARE AND HOME PRODUCTS

WHY

Many products used on our bodies and in our home contain toxic, heavy metals and other endocrine-disrupting chemicals that can enter through the lungs and skin.

- The accumulation from repeated daily use increases our toxic load and can damage our gut microbiome.
- Harsh cleaners and antibacterial soaps not only irritate our skin, they play a role in eliminating the good bacteria for our microbiome as a whole.

IDEAS FOR ACTION

- [ ] Swap out cleaning and personal care products made with parabens, artificial fragrances/phthalates.
- [ ] Avoid harsh soaps and shampoos with sodium lauryl sulfate.
- [ ] Use nail polish without triphenyl phosphate (TPHP).
- [ ] Use lead-free lipstick.
- [ ] Choose aluminum-free deodorant.
- [ ] Stop using antimicrobial products for non-acute situations (especially if made with triclosan).
- [ ] If budget is an issue, start with products that cover the most surface area (e.g. body lotion) and have the biggest risk (e.g. phthalates in fragrances and triclosan).

- ☐ Purchase cloth (linen, cotton or hemp) shower curtains or plastic versions made from PEVA (polyethylene vinyl acetate) rather than PVC.

- ☐ Try products like coconut oil and shea butter for moisturizers and lip balm.

- ☐ Look for non-toxic stain protectors and removers.

- ☐ Get rid of old, crumpling paint carefully and purchase lead-free, low VOC-paint when repainting.

- ☐ Switch to an organic mattress if possible.

- ☐ Get immediate professional help if you suspect mold in your home.

FOR MORE GUIDANCE

Toolkit: "Product Labels"; shellymalone.com/inflamed: "Favorite Products"

GOAL 15:
UPGRADE COOKWARE AND STORAGE CONTAINERS

WHY

Your clean, anti-inflammatory meals will likely be derailed if chemicals from your non-stick pan are leaching into it. The same goes for microwaving leftovers in BPA, phthalate-laden plastic containers.

- Non-stick pans can release carcinogenic perflourochemicals (PFCs), especially if the pan becomes scratched or you are cooking at high heats.

- Storing food — and especially reheating food — in plastic containers, can release endocrine disruptors, carcinogens, and other inflammatory materials.

IDEAS FOR ACTION

- [ ] Swap out plastic food containers for glass.

- [ ] Stop drinking out of plastic coffee lids — take them off or buy a BPA-free reusable cup (ideally stainless steel).

- [ ] Swap out non-stick cookware with stainless steel, cast iron or non-toxic ceramic pan. If budget is an issue, start with your most commonly used pan and work from there.

- [ ] Watch for (and avoid) plastics with polycarbonate, marked with a “PC” or “#7.”

GOAL 16:
COOK MORE

WHY

When we cook our own food, we take control over which ingredients we let into our bodies and which chemicals we don't. We may be able to avoid food sensitivities, but when eating packaged food or food we don't prepare ourselves, the quality of the other ingredients isn't always known (e.g. types of oils used, where the meat was sourced, quality of the produce or additives used).

IDEAS FOR ACTION

- ☐ Schedule into your calendar specific days and times of the week when you will: 1) plan your meals, 2) prepare your grocery list, 3) shop and prep food.
- ☐ Plan your meals for a week (or one day if that is where you need to start).
- ☐ Find a few staple recipes for breakfast, lunch and dinner that you won't mind repeating.
- ☐ Try 1 new recipe per week. If it goes over well, double it next time and freeze half.
- ☐ Take a whole food cooking class.
- ☐ If grocery shopping is a challenge, try grocery delivery services and join a CSA for local produce.
- ☐ If it is all too overwhelming, use a whole food meal delivery service that can accommodate special diets — either ready to eat or prepped and portioned for you to whip up

yourself. (The cost just might be off-set by food waste from poor planning…or medical bills).

FOR MORE GUIDANCE

Toolkit: "Recipe Resources," "Easy Dishes," "Pantry Staples to Stock"; shellymalone.com/inflamed: "Whole Food Delivery"

GOAL 17:
CONSUME INFLAMMATION-FIGHTING FOODS

WHY

We take an offensive stance and fight inflammation head on when we consume specific foods and herbs that have powerful anti-inflammatory properties. Integrating these into your daily or weekly meal plans can help you get in front of your pain or other symptoms of inflammation.

IDEAS FOR ACTION

- ☐ Frequently eat dishes with curry (or curcumin) and ginger, make a curry/ginger tea, or take a curcumin supplement (check with your physician if on blood-thinning medication).

- ☐ Make a daily smoothie that includes green Lacinato kale, blueberries, soaked walnuts, chia seeds and/or flaxseeds.

- ☐ Incorporate other inflammation-fighting foods into your diet including ginger, green leafy vegetables, tomatoes, cherries, olive oil, nuts (especially almonds and walnuts), and omega-3 fats like fatty fish, chia and flax seeds, and grass-fed beef, bison and pastured eggs.

FOR MORE GUIDANCE

Toolkit: "Pantry Staples to Stock," "Recipe Resources," "Which Fats When"

GOAL 18:
REST YOUR BODY

WHY

Constantly battling inflammation in and of itself is a huge source of fatigue. A lack of sleep (especially during strategic hours for your circadian rhythm) and overworking your body not only adds to this exhaustion, it causes more inflammation.

IDEAS FOR ACTION

- ☐ Be asleep no later than 11pm (before you get a second wind that can keep you up all night), with 10pm being ideal. Get at least 7 hours of sleep per night, aiming for 8.
  - ☐ Turn off all electronics at least 30 minutes before bedtime (ideally two hours) and don't keep them in your bedroom.
  - ☐ Avoid caffeine six hours prior to bedtime.
  - ☐ Use lavender bath salts or lavender essential oil before bedtime (put oil in an aromatherapy diffuser or put a few drops in a tissue and tuck under your pillow).
  - ☐ Keep a journal by your bed to note tasks to do the next day.
  - ☐ Try GABA (gamma aminobutyric acid) or short-term melatonin supplementation or acupuncture if you have persistent issues with sleeplessness.
  - ☐ Avoid alcohol. While it may help you *get* to sleep, it will disrupt your sleep through the night.

- ☐ Balance your workout routine.
    - ☐ If you have signs of over training (difficulty recovering, not losing weight/inches despite increased exercise), swap intense cardio or lifting sessions with a restorative yoga class or brisk walk a few days a week.
    - ☐ If you are not exercising at all, add in a 30-minute walk 3–5 times per week.

GOAL 19:
FREE YOUR MIND

WHY

Rest isn't only about your body, it's about your mind as well. If you're enduring chronic stress — constant issues at work, family angst, holding on to past resentments, living with unhealthy relationships, or ignoring your dreams and passions — you can bet it is having a significant effect on your immune system. If it continues, it will ultimately manifest an illness (if it hasn't already).

IDEAS FOR ACTION

- [ ] Find personal help in the form of a therapist or spiritual leader.
- [ ] Find an author or speaker that resonates with you and read/listen to their work regularly.
- [ ] Start a meditation or yoga practice (as little as 2 minutes a day can help).
- [ ] Get outside every day and spend time in whatever type of nature you can find.
- [ ] Spend more time with friends and family.
- [ ] Spend some time discovering your passions and do a little bit of that every day. Some helpful questions:
    - "If I was on my death bed right now, what would I regret not doing?"
    - "What work would I do for free?"
    - "What am I doing when time passes effortlessly?

- [ ] Consider GABA (gamma aminobutyric acid) supplementation or acupuncture for anxiety.

- [ ] Take another look at your *Why* and take steps towards being able to leave the office early, hire some help, and/or separate from any drama that is bringing you down.

FOR MORE GUIDANCE

Toolkit: "Mind Body Resources"

GOAL 20:
REDUCE YOUR CAFFEINE INTAKE

WHY

When you consume coffee, sodas, or energy drinks with a high caffeine content, your stress hormones (catecholamines) are increased, which can cause spikes in blood sugar. This results in corresponding spikes of insulin which then increases inflammation. Ultimately, you feel even more drained because you are taxing your adrenal glands, which play a vital role in your energy and stress response.

IDEAS FOR ACTION

- [ ] If giving up coffee is an absolute non-starter for you, take it down to one cup of organic coffee per day, as coffee bean crops are heavily sprayed with pesticides.

- [ ] Introduce white, green, or other herbal tea into your day instead of a second (or third) cup of coffee.

- [ ] Swap carbonated soda for kombucha, mineral water or club soda.

- [ ] Make it your overall goal to get down to just one caffeinated beverage each day, while eliminating energy drinks and soda altogether.

FOR MORE GUIDANCE

shellymalone.com/inflamed: “Favorite Products”

GOAL 21:
REDUCE ALCOHOL

WHY

Alcohol not only will affect the quality of your sleep, excessive amounts can have serious health consequences. Chronic alcohol use will:

- impair detoxification and can lead to a leaky gut
- create blood sugar imbalances and inflammatory insulin spikes
- increase the risk of breast cancer in women

Not to mention, suffering from a hangover leads to sugar cravings and poor food choices.

IDEAS FOR ACTION

- ☐ Work towards limiting alcohol to three or less drinks per week.
- ☐ Choose red wine over white wine (ideally organic).
- ☐ Choose any wine over liquor or sugary mixed drinks.
- ☐ Choose tequila or clear alcohol (e.g. grape-based vodka), over dark alcohol.
- ☐ Incorporate an every other approach, drinking sparkling water or club soda in between cocktails to help you limit quantities consumed.

GOAL 22:
STOP SMOKING COMPLETELY

WHY

Smoking can cause cancer to almost any part of your body, as well as systemic inflammation. There is no safe amount of smoking. Cigarettes may be more addictive than heroin and cocaine so even occasional or social smoking can lead to regular use.

IDEAS FOR ACTION

- [ ] Take a long hard look at your *Why.* Write it down and read it every day (or every minute if you need to).
- [ ] Seek professional help or outside support to understand the underlying reasons for smoking.
- [ ] See a professional practitioner that can provide natural therapies, amino acids or other supplementation to address addiction and any underlying depression.
- [ ] Eat to combat any underlying depression: consume pasture-raised animal protein for tryptophan (the precursor to the neurotransmitter serotonin), omega-3 fats, a variety of fresh fruits and vegetables.

FOR MORE GUIDANCE

Toolkit: "Finding a Progressive Practitioner"; CDC "Guide for Quitting Smoking" and mobile app

GOAL 23:
REDUCE NSAID USE, WHEN POSSIBLE

WHY

I can't (and won't) interfere with any specific medical treatment plan you are following, but I can encourage you to focus on the root cause of your issues. It is well-supported in research that this class of pain relievers causes damage to your digestive tract, and that similar relief of pain and inflammation can be seen with natural alternatives.

IDEAS FOR ACTION

- [ ] For chronic aches and pains, seek out physical therapy, acupuncture or osteopathy. Use ice or heat to alleviate pain if possible.
- [ ] Consider turmeric and cod liver oil supplements.
- [ ] Look into food sensitivities (including food additives) for joint pain or other chronic pain.
- [ ] Increase the amount and variety of your fruit and vegetables to increase your antioxidant intake.
- [ ] Limit the stress in your life and ensure adequate water intake to help with chronic headaches.

FOR MORE GUIDANCE

Toolkit: "Find a Progressive Practitioner"; shellymalone.com/inflamed: "Elimination Diet Template"

GOAL 24:
SUPPLEMENT (APPROPRIATELY)

WHY

It is ideal to get all required nutrients from your diet. There is a food synergy that comes from consuming nutrients in their whole form that isn't received from isolated, synthetic supplements. However, nutrient deficiencies are common with inflammation and disease, so supplementation will likely be needed for your healing. There are common supplements that are likely safe and of benefit to everyone with chronic inflammation. Beyond that, it is best to work with a qualified practitioner to customize a supplement regime because:

- the nature of the conditions you may be suffering from — and the treatment of them — can vary greatly.
- there is potential for drug-supplement or supplement-supplement interactions.
- your current nutrient status, genetics and biochemistry are very individual.

IDEAS FOR ACTION

Start with a daily supplementation of:

- ☐ Cod liver oil for important fat-soluble vitamins — A and D — in addition to inflammation fighting omega-3 fatty acids (check with your physician is you are taking blood thinning or antihypertensive medications).
- ☐ A multi-strain probiotic/day (10–25 billion CFU's) that includes lactobacillus and bifidobacterium; if you have yeast (candida) it should only contain the strain, *Saccharomyces boulardi.*

- [ ] A whole food multivitamin capsule (gluten-free, non-GMO).

Other supplements to discuss with your practitioner:

- [ ] Gut healing: L-glutamine, zinc, marshmallow root, slippery elm (not for anyone following a specific carbohydrate diet)
- [ ] Anti-inflammatories: boswellia, quercetin, aloe vera juice, turmeric, alpha-lipoic acid, curcumin, vitamin D, coenzyme Q10
- [ ] Antioxidants/Detoxification: vitamins A, C, E, selenium, glutathione
- [ ] Digestive aids: digestive enzymes, HCL, or apple cider vinegar

FOR MORE GUIDANCE

Toolkit: "Find a Progressive Practitioner"

As noted in Goal 13: If you have been diagnosed with SIBO or an intolerance to histamines or FODMAPS — or suspect you may have any of these conditions — do not start probiotics without first consulting with a qualified health practitioner familiar with digestive health.

GOAL 25:
WORK WITH A PROGRESSIVE PROFESSIONAL

WHY

Not only can a professional, licensed practitioner help you with an individualized supplementation plan, they can ensure the proper testing is done to identify underlying causes of inflammation and an appropriate treatment plan based on your individual needs.

The key is to find someone progressive-minded — ideally trained in integrative and functional medicine — that will focus on the root cause of your symptoms and not rely only on pharmaceutical symptom management.

IDEAS FOR ACTION

- ☐ Check with your insurance to find out your benefits for nutrition counseling, out-of-network and integrative/functional practitioners. Many practitioners in this area will not take insurance, but you should be eligible for some amount of reimbursement.

- ☐ Make a plan to budget for the services if this will be a financial burden, keeping in mind there is money to be saved in long-term better health.

- ☐ Locate an appropriate licensed practitioner in your area. Ideally, look for a physician trained in integrative or functional medicine who works with a registered dietitian nutritionist or other licensed nutrition professional.

- ☐ Work with a biological dentist to have any mercury amalgams removed safely.

- [ ] Talk to your practitioner about assessing: micronutrient status, food sensitivities, genetic variations (especially the MTHFR variation), hormone levels, heavy metal levels, hidden infections.

FOR MORE GUIDANCE

Toolkit: "Find a Progressive Practitioner"

BALANCING WHAT'S IDEAL WITH WHAT'S REAL

You are now ready to put your personal plan into action.

But before you do, I want to acknowledge that we are all actual humans. Remember, I suggested one change every two weeks. You shouldn't put undue pressure on yourself to incorporate all of the above suggestions in one fell swoop (unless you are extremely motivated, and then absolutely "lean in" my friend). So if you are very resistant, overwhelmed with a new diagnosis (or with the resulting symptoms), or the current mainstays of your diet are frozen pizza and cheeseburgers, then just take a deep breath. Choose one new goal now. And in a couple of weeks, choose another. Know that slow and steady can still win the race, all you have to do is take one baby step forward and you're in it.

And speaking of babies, you should know I've got a couple of them, one of which is a 3-year-old boy. I'm confident he has a successful career in the WWF ahead of him. I have about 30 seconds to prep meals before that guy scales the wall and jumps in the oven. And he's about as helpful as a pet goat in the grocery store. Kid wrangling, working and traveling also don't lend themselves to always getting the rest I need, sticking with a consistent meditation practice, or exercise routine, so I get it. Life happens and when it does, sometimes a shortcut is the only way — and that's okay too.

I should also note that I'm 40. And, I'm as vain as the next girl. So make no mistake — I need skincare and cosmetics that WORK. Trust me when I say that heavy metals and endocrine disruptors are not requirements for products to be effective.

I've purposely provided simple resources in the Toolkit that aren't intimidating — very simple dishes and snacks, mobile apps to research products and implement mind-body practices, lists of specific products I use (available for download on my website, not paid endorsements). No matter what road blocks you may be facing, know that there are easy solutions to ease you into this major lifestyle change. And if you have a need to go deeper, I have options for that too — recipe books and websites and recommendations for further reading.

If you're concerned about living a life of deprivation, take comfort in these honest words: I love the food I eat and do not miss my previous gluten- and dairy-laden meals. In fact, my new way of eating has broadened the palate of this self-proclaimed "super taster" who didn't even try a tomato until college. Not to mention, jumping off the calorie- and fat-counting crazy train allowed me to welcome in formerly restricted foods like avocados, (pastured) butter, nuts and high-quality meats — other than a skinless chicken breast. My sweet tooth is virtually gone and over time I naturally evolved into someone who eats more consciously.

THE ROAD I'M (STILL) TRAVELING

My journey to a completely whole, anti-inflammatory lifestyle is still in progress, and to be totally honest, I'm not sure if I'll ever get there (although my chances increase — I hope — once both kids are older than 10). I started with taking out foods I was sensitive to, primarily gluten, dairy, corn, and soy. Thankfully, I received such an immediate relief of my symptoms, I was motivated to make that work however I could. While I did eat mostly organic and non-GMO, I didn't care if that food came from a can, a plastic bag, or the freezer, because not only was I new to this way of eating, I was a new mom, too.

Over time, I've worked on balancing the other side — more good fats, a lot more vegetables, and more fermented foods. I'm cooking whole foods more, but there is still a lot of room for improvement. I'm extremely lucky to live in a community where I have a lot of very healthy dining and on-the-go options, so I take full advantage of that. But, I have also taken whole foods cooking classes and I still research recipes that sound like they might work for my family.

Finding balance in my life and managing my stress is something I constantly strive for. In the Toolkit I have a list of recommended reading about spiritual approaches I've used that have been life-changing for me. But, what first took me out of my victim mentality about my diagnosis, and ultimately helped me with chronic anxiety that kept me constantly under stress was this simple concept: being present.

I know saying "live in the now" sounds so cliché, but it's more true and farther reaching than most people realize. No one breaks it down better for me than Eckhart Tolle in *The Power of Now.* He challenges the "life-corroding insanity" of our resistance to the present moment, and eloquently explains that allowing an internal fight between living "here" but wanting to be "there" is what causes our stress and anxiety. Having friends and family who deal with the same split focus and panic over the unknown doesn't make the struggle any less crazy. When we fully accept this very moment, and release future "what if's," it allows us to settle down and have faith that the answers we are looking for will be there when we need them.

In my efforts to stay present and do what's right for me and my body, I have a spiritual practice, but I struggle to stick with it every single day. My consistency with exercise ebbs and flows with my workload. I'm very discerning with the ingredients I put on and in my body, but that doesn't mean I won't enjoy a green salad at a dinner party because it may not be organic.

Perfection isn't the goal—feeling better is. One step at a time. Use the Toolkit and guidance from this book to learn from your mistakes and find a better way to live.

EPILOGUE

BEING YOUR OWN ADVOCATE

Up until my RA diagnosis, my educational and professional backgrounds were as conventional as could be. And to be honest, I battled with my own ego to accept that these progressive nutrition interventions — ones that in all my years of study were unknown to me — were providing me (and many others, I quickly learned) dramatic results.

My diagnosis morphed me into a living, breathing product of a system that puts the onus on the patient to become educated, consult with multiple specialists, ask the tough questions, decipher the differing opinions and ultimately advocate for themselves for the course of treatment that they believe is best for them.

While I have the utmost respect for many of our medical innovations and the clinicians who execute them, when it comes to the treatment (or prevention) of chronic conditions, the overall approach of the Western-bent medical community leaves something to be desired. Ideally, we wouldn't treat symptoms by loading up on medications, we would instead focus energy on discovering the root causes of those symptoms and put efforts towards prevention.

During my first days of my master's program for public health, a simple, powerful parable was shared with me by one of my professors. It not only left a lasting impression, it has directed my perspective ever since:

> Imagine a large river with a bridge going across the top of it. At the end of this river dozens of people are working frantically to fix the injuries of those who have fallen in. As the people along the shore are trying to treat and rescue as many as possible one woman looks up and sees a seemingly never-ending stream of people falling through the bridge and begins to run upstream. One of other rescuers screams angrily, "Where are you going? There are so many people that need help here." To which the woman replied, "I'm going upstream to fix the bridge."

This timeless anecdote exemplifies for me the differing sensibilities between more progressive (a.k.a. integrative, functional, holistic, complementary) care, which looks to find and resolve the root cause of an issue, and conventional (aka allopathic, Western) care, which aims to patch you up with a shiny bandage.

In my experience, both as a practitioner and a patient, conventional medicine can be quite incredulous and sometimes cavalier about the critical role lifestyle plays in health and healing, and can have a skewed view towards treatment over prevention. And when the nutrition and lifestyle principles being discussed are not as mainstream, the heels are really dug in.

However, early on in my professional career, I was taught that it's never the person but the process that is to blame for inadequacies or poor outcomes in any situation. And I think that principle is quite fitting here. It is our healthcare system as a whole that prevents adaptation to new principles.

Inflamed is not filled with radical ideas about how conventional medicine and the government are in cahoots to sabotage our good health. However, I am encouraging you to think critically about what drives the business of food and nutrition, and the larger health system. Think about how what goes on behind the scenes may affect not only the information you get from your providers and the mainstream media, but the care that those conventional medicine practitioners are able to provide.

Our current healthcare system is so bogged down by bureaucracy that they cannot make quick changes or respond to new research. In fact, even after solid research has been completed and proven a new treatment to be significantly effective, it takes an average of 17 years to become standard of care. The more progressive practice is far more agile and innovative as it's not held down by the same red tape and protocol. However, while a more effective long-term outcome could be your result while working outside the mainstream, the services of a progressive practitioner are available only to those who can afford to pay out-of-pocket, as these services aren't always covered by insurance. A heartbreaking disparity in access to care.

So in an effort to understand your healthcare options, we have to advocate for ourselves and look beyond just what's offered and into why.

FINDING THE BETTER WAY

The concepts in this book have a pretty low risk profile. This isn't an extreme diet — I'm not suggesting you starve, avoid solid food, or drink cyanide. This is all about altering lifestyle and your food choices and coming away from the pitiful standard American diet (SAD) that leaves us overfed and undernourished. The U.S. is ranked 37th in health globally and North America has the highest prevalence of obesity. So bucking the norm (when the norm kind of sucks) seems like a pretty good call.

But lifelong, consistent change is not easy. You must find that deeper answer to make it worth taking these steps toward improved health. You need to discover your personal *Why.*

I can't give you your answer. But, I can share mine.

I was driven to change because I wanted to have the energy to enjoy my newborn daughter. To decrease the pain in my hands so that I could hold and feed her again. It was my desire to compete again in beach volleyball, and to enjoy all the other physical activities that had been such a huge part of my life. To avoid inundating my body and enduring the nasty side effects of the drugs I was about to be prescribed.

And I was determined to let faith replace fear. I wanted to believe that I would enjoy a healthful future. I couldn't fully live my life if I was scared of ending up in the wheelchair my first rheumatologist predicted could be in my future when he said there was no way to know how quickly my disease would progress.

If I couldn't wholeheartedly promote these dietary and lifestyle principles, I wouldn't have written this book.

So, if you're reading because you are searching for a new perspective, or if you just want a good dose of common sense to get you back on track, know that I walk the talk. My guess is that if you give this way of life a real chance, you will benefit in ways both recognizable and invisible. If you've been suffering, chances are your symptoms will wane. And if you don't have a specific issue you're dealing with, all the good, healthy, clean steps you're taking are potentially helping you avoid disease and other serious problems.

As Dr. Terry Wahls, a leading expert in autoimmunity, said, "May you never know what you might have prevented."

So looking forward, I hope you buy into this paradigm shift. I hope you find yourself more interested in the quality of your food and the effect certain foods have on your health, than you are in counting calories and fat grams. I hope you think critically about the stress your body endures on all levels — toxic chemicals, mental stress, lack of rest, and deficiencies in key nutrients that your body requires in order to run optimally.

Most of all, I hope you've found on these pages the answers you've been searching for — a reason and a way to get back your health, and a newfound belief in the power of an anti-inflammatory lifestyle.

PART FOUR
TOOLKIT

All of the guides in the Toolkit and more are available for download at shellymalone.com/inflamed

PANTRY STAPLES TO STOCK

PRODUCT	TO REPLACE
Basics	
Wide variety of organic produce (ideally local and seasonal). Frozen okay.	Conventional produce, especially those on the Environmental Working Group's (EWG) Dirty Dozen
Grass-fed or pastured, organic eggs and meat products; wild fish	Conventionally grown eggs and meat; farmed fish
Himalayan or Celtic sea salt	Table salt
Filtered water (reverse osmosis ideal)	Tap or non-filtered bottled water
Almond, coconut, hemp or cashew milk products If no sensitivity to casein: raw, organic, grass-fed WHOLE FAT goat, sheep, cow milk	Pasteurized, low-fat cow's milk products (milk, ice cream, yogurt, cheese…)

BECAUSE
• Reduce pesticides & avoid GMOs • Better nutrient value and flavor • Fresh produce provides inflammation-fighting antioxidants (esp. blueberries, beets, greens).

• Conventionally grown animals are:
  • given synthetic growth hormones & antibiotics
  • fed diets of GMO feed (mostly corn), rather than high omega-3, inflammation-fighting grass
  • farmed fish has higher levels of carcinogenic PCBs

• Minimal processing retains vital trace minerals — like magnesium and potassium — that assist your body in metabolizing the sodium. • Avoids exposure to chemicals used in processing regular table salt.
• Excess fluoride, other heavy metals and prescription medication waste can increase toxic load and disrupt thyroid hormones.
• Cow's milk is high in inflammatory A1 beta-casein. • Pasteurized, non-organic dairy products contain added growth hormones, antibiotics/steroids, are fed GMO corn & stripped of enzymes that help with digestion.

PRODUCT	TO REPLACE
Grains	
100% whole grain gluten-free oats and ancient grains (e.g. millet, quinoa, amaranth, almond), sweet rice (sorghum) flour Grain-free flours (coconut, almond, arrowroot)	Wheat-containing (or grain-containing) flour
Brown rice, or grain-free tortillas	Regular flour or corn tortillas, tortilla/corn chips
Gluten-free, or grain-free granola	Traditional versions made with conventionally processed oats (for cereal, parfait, snacks)
Baking	
Liquid oils: organic, cold-pressed extra virgin olive, palm, flax and/or avocado oil Solid oils: ghee, coconut oil, organic/grass-fed butter* and animal fats * only if/when determined you can tolerate casein.	Canola, peanut, corn, margarine or other processed vegetable oils that are inflammatory and can be from genetically-modified sources
Raw, organic honey; real maple syrup, molasses, Lakanto sugar, Stevia	Refined and/or artificial sweeteners

BECAUSE
• Wheat flour contains gluten, which can be inflammatory and damage intestinal lining. • Some individuals need to avoid all grains.
Flour tortillas contain wheat and corn tortillas are likely GMO (unless specifically stated otherwise).
Unless certified gluten-free, oats are processed with wheat and can be contaminated with gluten.
Organic = no pesticides or GMOs Cold-pressed = retaining vital nutrients and flavor Extra-virgin = minimally processed (and a more delicate flavor) Grass-fed = high omega-3 from animals eating grass instead of corn
• Refined sugar is harmful to entire system and could have GMOs • Artificial sweeteners are made of chemicals toxic to your system • Stevia/Lakanto sugar have zero glycemic index

PRODUCT	TO REPLACE
Spices/Condiments	
Fresh or dried herbs/natural seasonings (cloves, turmeric, ginger & rosemary, garlic)	Processed seasonings with artificial preservatives
Organic, wheat-free tamari or liquid aminos; coconut liquid aminos	Soy sauce
Organic ketchup and mustards	Conventional condiments
Non-GMO, soy-free mayo	Conventional mayo
Almond butter	Conventional peanut butter
Beverages	
Mineral water	Soda, diet soda, energy drinks
White/green tea	Coffee
Kombucha	Soda, juice
Coconut water	Traditional sports drinks, pasteurized fruit juice

BECAUSE
• Processed seasonings contain many food additives (e.g. MSG) • May contain gluten • Particular spices are powerful anti-inflammatories
• Soy sauce contains wheat • Tamari does not contain wheat, but contains soy. Organic versions will ensure it is non-GMO. • Coconut aminos are gluten- and soy-free.
• Conventional condiments are almost always made with corn syrup or high fructose corn syrup and additives.
• Conventional mayo can contain GMOs, soy, processed oils, cow's milk and artificial ingredients.
• Peanuts have a toxin in them that make them hard to tolerate for many and most conventional brands have refined sugar & artificial ingredients.
• Avoid excess processed sugar and harmful chemicals.
• High in polyphenols, much lower in cortisol-increasing caffeine. • Non-organic coffee beans are high in pesticides.
• Provides much needed probiotics that aid in gut health and immunity.
• Contains electrolytes without processed sugar/chemicals • For sports, hangovers, colds, headaches and any other time you need additional hydration.

GUIDE TO GMOS

GM CROPS IN PRODUCTION NOW	GM CROPS IN THE QUEUE
Alfalfa	White Russet Potato
Canola	Rice
Corn	Salmon
Cotton	Pigs
Papaya	
Soy	
Sugar beets	
Zucchini & Yellow Summer Squash	

Ingredients that could be derived from GMOs: Amino Acids, Aspartame, Ascorbic Acid, Sodium Ascorbate, Vitamin C, Citric Acid, Sodium Citrate, Ethanol, Flavorings (natural and artificial), High-Fructose Corn Syrup, Hydrolyzed Vegetable Protein, Lactic Acid, Maltodextrins, Molasses, Monosodium Glutamate (MSG), Sucrose, Textured Vegetable Protein (TVP), Xanthan Gum, Some Vitamins, Yeast Products

GUIDE TO ORGANIC

LEAST HARMFUL – LOWEST AMOUNT OF PESTICIDES	MOST HARMFUL – HIGHEST AMOUNT OF PESTICIDES
Avocado	Apples
Pineapple	Peaches
Cabbage	Nectarines
Sweet Peas (frozen)	Strawberries
Onions	Grapes
Asparagus	Celery
Mangoes	Spianch
Papaya	Sweet Bell Peppers
Kiwi	Cucumbers
Eggplant	Cherry Tomatoes
Grapefruit	Snap Peas (Imported)
Cantaloupe	Potatoes
Cauliflower	Hot Peppers
Sweet Potatoes	Kale/Collard Greens

The Environmental Working Group Consumer Guides for "Genetically Modified Food" and "EWG's Shopper's Guides to Pesticides in Produce"

WHICH FATS WHEN

Note: All animal fats should be from pastured or grass-fed, organic and/or hormone-free sources

FATS TO USE

Baking	Non-Heated/Salad Dressing
Ghee (clarified butter – no casein)	Cold-pressed, extra-virgin olive oil
Butter (if casein is tolerated)	Avocado oil
Coconut oil	Walnut oil
Rendered lard	
Cooking	**Whole Foods**
Ghee	Avocado
Butter	Nuts (especially walnuts, almonds, pecans and macadamia)
Coconut oil	Seeds (especially sesame, chia, pumpkin, hemp)
Non-hydrogenated palm oil	Wild, fatty fish or cod liver oil supplements
Rendered tallow, lard, or poultry fat	Pastured eggs

FATS TO AVOID

Hydrogenated or partially hydrogenated oil, margarine, corn oil, soybean oil, cottonseed oil, peanut oil, safflower oil, canola oil

EASY DISHES

BREAKFAST

Pastured eggs with sautéed vegetables (scramble, omelet, frittata) topped with avocado and/or fermented hot sauce

Avocado toast (on whole-grain, gluten-free or grain-free bread)

Soaked, gluten-free oats or other ancient grain, or a grain-free granola

Pastured/grass-fed, organic, hormone-free, nitrate-free chicken or turkey sausage/bacon

Parfait: Dairy-free yogurt, fruit, gluten-free granola, drizzle of honey, sprinkle of bee pollen

Whole grain, gluten-free, and/or grain-free pancakes or waffles with almond butter or pastured butter and real maple syrup

Smoothies (fruit, kale, almond/hemp/cashew milk, soaked walnuts, coconut oil or almond butter, bee pollen)

LUNCH/DINNER ITEMS

Green salad with small amount of animal protein, nuts or seeds, avocado, olive oil-based dressing

Wild tuna salad or organic chicken salad (see Mayo options in 'Favorite Products' list). Enjoy as an open-faced, gluten-free sandwich, on a bed of greens, or solo. Option to add some diced kimchi in salad.

Open-faced sandwich with nitrate-free lunchmeat (ideally whole, unprocessed meat) with greens, avocado, tomato, sprouts and sauerkraut

Grilled wild salmon or salmon patties

Fajitas or tacos on non-GMO corn tortillas (if a corn sensitivity has been ruled out) or a grain-free tortilla

Grass-fed burgers or turkey/beef/bison meatballs with mustard sauce

Sweet potato, yucca or zucchini fries

Baked or whipped sweet potatoes

Sautéed greens (lacinato kale, Swiss chard, collard greens) or baked vegetables in coconut or olive oil with lemon, garlic and sea salt

EASY ON-THE-GO SNACKS

Organic apples, bananas or celery with almond/cashew butter

Hummus or tahini & carrots (or any other cut-up veggies you can find....or with gluten-free crackers/pretzels)

Hard-boiled egg

Gluten-free, dairy-free, non-GMO energy bars

Kale chips (drizzle with olive oil, sprinkle with sea salt and bake at 350 for 10-15 minutes)

Parfait – coconut or almond yogurt topped with fruit, a sprinkle of gluten-free granola, raw honey and a sprinkle of bee pollen

Smoothie – non-dairy milk, frozen berries, kale, walnuts, chia seed, coconut oil, bee pollen

Trail mix – make your own with favorite nuts/seeds, dairy-free chocolate chips, dark chocolate chips/chunks or cacao nibs, dried fruit (raisins, dried cranberries, currants, etc.).

Raw nuts – anything other than peanuts

Avocado

Unsulphured, unsweetened dried mango (or other fruit)

Certified gluten-free, or grain-free granola

Coconut or almond yogurt

Sweet potato, or other root vegetable, chips

Non-GMO popcorn (only if a corn sensitivity has been ruled out)

Grass-fed jerky

RECIPE RESOURCES

PAMELA SALZMAN

pamelasalzman.com, Instagram: @pamelasalzman.

Delicious, whole-food recipes that accommodate many food sensitivities. Cooking classes in Los Angeles and weekly meal plan ideas also available.

SPROUTED KITCHEN

sproutedkitchen.com; *A Tastier Take on Whole Foods* cookbook

AGAINST ALL GRAIN

Against All Grain Meals Made Easy Cookbook; Cookery mobile app

PRODUCT LABELS

LABELS TO LOOK FOR:	LABELS TO LOOK OUT FOR:
Animal Products:	
Organic, Pastured, Pasture-Raised, 100% Grass-Fed and Grass-Finished (even with a grass-fed label, animals could be grain-finished), Wild, Nitrate-Free/No Nitrates Added, Antibiotic-Free, Hormone-Free	Vegetarian-Fed (could be GMO corn feed), Cage-Free and Free-Range (for eggs – they are corn-fed and still have little room to roam)
Packaged Foods:	
No Artificial Colors, No Artificial Flavors, No Artificial Sweeteners, Non-GMO, Certified Gluten-Free*, Dairy-Free, Soy-Free	Sugar-Free/Low-Calorie (likely has artificial sweeteners), Low-Fat (could have added sugars), Natural (no clear standard)
Personal Care Products	
Paraben-Free, Phthalate-Free, BPA-Free, Fragrance-Free, Sodium Lauryl Sulfate- (or SLS) free, PABA-Free (sunscreen), TPHP-/ Formaldehyde-/Toluene-Free (nail polish)	Natural or Non-Toxic (no clear standard), Hypoallergenic or Dermatologist-tested (could still contain endocrine disruptors)

*not necessary for whole foods naturally gluten-free: fruits and vegetables, nuts, water, meat, rice, etc.

HELPFUL TOOLS FOR PRODUCT LABELS

Environmental Working Groups (EWG) Consumer Guides: "Food Scores," "EWG's Skin Deep Guide to Cosmetics"

EWG's Healthy Living mobile app (search or scan bar code to check safety of specific food and personal care products)

NAVIGATING GLUTEN

GRAINS WITH GLUTEN	GRAINS/FLOURS WITHOUT GLUTEN
Wheat, Rye, *Spelt, Kamut, Barley, Triticale, Oats (unless certified gluten-free), **Farro, **Einkorn, **Emmer, Couscous	Rice, Potato/Sweet Potato/ Yams, Quinoa, *Buckwheat, Amaranth, Sorghum, Millet, Teff, Tapioca, Nut Flours, Bean Flours, Coconut Flour

*does not contain wheat, but does contain gluten
**considered lower in gluten, but are not gluten-free

OTHER/HIDDEN SOURCES OF GLUTEN

Any baked or other goods made with flours from gluten-containing grains mentioned above

Fried foods (unless specified otherwise, e.g. French fries not dusted with wheat flour)

Soy sauce (unless specified wheat-free, like tamari)

Artificial crab (used in most sushi California rolls, unless you specify "real" or "King" crab), some sticky sushi rice

Some salad dressings or sauces (e.g. Worcestershire sauce, teriyaki sauce)

Some processed meats (e.g. sausage, pepperoni, lunch meats)

Flavorings and additives (e.g. MSG, hydrolyzed vegetable proteins, malt)

Beer (unless specifically stated "gluten-free")

Some nutritional supplements and medications

NAVIGATING DAIRY

DAIRY PRODUCTS WITH CASEIN	DAIRY PRODUCTS WITHOUT CASEIN
Following products from any animal: milk, cheese, yogurt, ice cream, butter, kefir	Eggs, almond and other nut milks, coconut milk, hemp milk, ghee (clarified butter)

CASEIN TOLERANCE (FROM MOST TOLERATED TO LEAST)

Raw goat or sheep milk products

Raw A2 cow's milk from Jersey or Guernsey cows (specifically bred for A2 casein)

Raw cow milk from standard A1 casein Holstein cows

Pasteurized, grass-fed, organic cow milk

Pasteurized, conventional (not grass-fed or organic) cow milk

Note: Butter can sometimes be tolerated because it is primarily fat, with very little casein protein. Kefir and some yogurts can also sometimes be tolerable because the fermentation helps break down the casein.

HIGH FODMAP FOODS

FRUIT	
Apples	Nectarines
Apricots	Peaches
Avocados	Pears
Blackberries	Persimmon
Cherries	Plums
Lychees	Prunes
Mangoes	Watermelon
VEGETABLES	
Artichokes	Cauliflower
Asparagus	Green Onion (bulb)
Beets	Leeks
Brussel Sprouts	Mushrooms
Cabbage	Onion

GRAINS/STARCHES /LEGUMES	
All Legumes	Sugar Snap Peas
Snow Peas	Wheat
SWEETENERS	
Agave	High Fructose Corn Syrup
Corn Syrup	Honey
Fructose	Sugar Alcohols (sorbitol, xylitol, mannitol, maltitol)
LACTOSE	
All milk	Soft cheese
Cream	Yogurt
TEA	
Chicory Tea	Dandelion Tea

LESSER EVILS

You Want This:	In an Ideal World:
Dairy (milk, cheese, yogurt, ice cream, etc.)	Avoid altogether. Choose almond, cashew, coconut, rice or hemp alternatives. NOTE: If you haven't ruled out a casein sensitivity, you must stay strictly dairy-free
Soda	Avoid completely. Choose properly filtered water, or iced herbal tea.
Snacks (potato chips, fries, etc.)	Avoid all fried foods, refined starches (e.g. white potatoes, potato starch), and refined oils. Choose homemade root vegetable chips or sweet potato fries, raw nuts or gluten-free granola.
Sweets	Avoid – conquer sugar cravings. Make your own cleaner versions using gluten- or grain-free flours, natural sweeteners, or swap with dark chocolate (at least 70% cocoa).
Bread	Only 100% whole grain, non-GMO, gluten-free (or grainless) made from scratch or a trusted bakery without additives. If confirmed not gluten sensitive, sprouted wheat bread.

When Your World is More Real than Ideal:	At The Very Least, Seek Out:
Raw, organic, grass fed goat/sheep milk; raw cow's milk, fermented kefir (less casein and/or retains enzymes that aid in digestion).	Organic preferred. At a minimum rBST-free and take a digestive enzyme 20 minutes before consumption.
Mineral water, club soda, kombucha	Black tea, natural sodas with no artificial sweeteners or corn syrup
Roasted, but otherwise whole nuts unsalted or with sea salt, rice/ancient grain crackers, purchased sweet potato fries (ensuring they aren't dusted with wheat flour), non-GMO natural potato chips	Packaged nuts (may be packed in refined oils and added salt), non-GMO corn chips or popcorn
Dried fruit, quinoa cookies or other dairy/gluten-free options without refined sugar or additives	Packaged items that are gluten- & dairy-free
Ancient grain or whole grain that may be made with some refined starches or GMO-free corn, but still gluten- & dairy-free.	Gluten-free bread products

BUDGETING IDEAS

- Plan meals ahead of time to reduce waste.
- Cook as much as possible to save on packaged goods.
- Eat whole, naturally gluten-free foods. Gluten-free packaged goods are typically more expensive.
- Pick one or two packaged items that you or your family consume regularly and make from scratch.
- Join thrivemarket.com and look into their THRIVE Gives program.
- Use frozen, organic fruits and vegetables.
- Join a CSA (community supported agriculture) to save money on fresh, local, organic, seasonal produce.
- Grow your own fruits, vegetables and herbs.
- Go in with friends or family and purchase an entire pastured cow (you'll need a big freezer) or join a meat CSA.

FIND A PROGRESSIVE PRACTITIONER

Institute of Functional Medicine

Dietitians in Integrative and Functional Medicine

American Association of Naturopathic Physicians

Holistic Dental Association

Dawn DeSylvia, MD, Integrative Family Practice
Website: drdesylvia.com
Office Tel: 310-914-3400
Email: info@wholelifehealthmd.com

A board certified family medicine physician who served on faculty at UCLA, Dr. Desylvia brings over 15 years of experience in Complementary and Alternative Medicine. At her Integrative Functional Medicine Center — Whole Life Health — she works with patients to identify the specific sources of their inflammation in order to both prevent and treat disease.

Note: this is not an all-inclusive list. The important thing is to find a licensed practitioner that you trust and works within a methodology (e.g. integrative, functional, holistic) that focuses on the root cause of the issue.

MIND-BODY RESOURCES

BOOKS

The Power of Now and *A New Earth* by Eckhart Tolle

A Return to Love and *A Year of Miracles* by Marianne Williamson

Miracles Now: 108 Life-Changing Tools for Less Stress, More Flow, and Finding Your True Purpose by Gabrielle Bernstein

The Untethered Soul by Michael A. Singer

TOOLS/WEBSITES

Headspace Mobile App (and website)

Happify™ Mobile App (and website)

Emotional Freedom Technique (EFT)

Promoting Positivity: 2-minute inspirational affirmations for health, happiness and more that you can download to your phone or mp3 player to listen to anywhere. http://www.promotingpositivity.com/

RECOMMENDED READING

The Omnivores Dilemma, Michael Pollan

The Microbiome Solution, Robynne Chutkan, MD

The Wahls Protocol, Dr. Terry Wahls (for autoimmune disease)

The Blood Sugar Solution, Mark Hyman, MD

The UltraMind Solution, Mark Hyman, MD

The Mood Cure, Julia Ross, M.A.

ACKNOWLEDGEMENTS

To be able to put this book into the world — the book I wanted and needed when I was first diagnosed with rheumatoid arthritis — is a gift I will always be grateful for. It would not have been possible without the support, guidance and love from so many.

My deepest gratitude to...

Amy Howard, my dear friend and hilarious human. Thank you for helping me to find my voice, and lending your brilliant Auto-Tune along the way. I could have never persevered through the final pushes without your years of support or your comic relief. I think we might have just started solids...

Marla Miller, for your guidance that refined my vision, and my voice. Your careful attention to my manuscript and the experience the reader should have gave clarity to my message. I am so grateful for our initial, fateful meeting.

Paula Page and Tolly Moseley at Paula Page PR, for taking on a little gal with a big plan. Working with you added joy to this project and your belief in me was critical in getting me to the finish line.

Heather Williams, my beautiful, magical friend. Thank you for keeping me focused on the deeper journey and helping me to find my "Big Magic." You are such a gift and I am so thankful that I've had you in my life for so many years.

Visionary doctors such as Mark Hyman, MD, Terry Wahls, MD and Chris Kresser, M.S., L.Ac who have so loudly advocated for the power of nutrition as both a means of prevention and a treatment for disease and provided credibility to progressive health methodologies.

My close friends who have always encouraged and supported me — Nicole, Debi, Amy, Micaela, Jen, Sharon and so many more. And a special thanks to those that endured my repeated harassment for market research and insight: Teale, Jen, Jess, Stephanie, Kendra, Rachel.

To those who I pretend are my friends, but most have no idea who I am — Marianne Williamson, Eckhart Tolle, the late Wayne Dyer, Elizabeth Gilbert, Jen Sincero, Marie Forleo — thank you for the inspiration and the tools you have provided me to get past the disillusionment of fear and discover what is really true.

James, for supporting me even when you didn't really get it. Thank you for dealing with the crazy that ensued to get this book out into the world and for your sacrifice. While the book is complete, I make no promises about the crazy.

My Mom, Sheri, for the unwavering support and selflessness you have showed me my entire life. Know that your fight only adds fuel to my fire to demand answers and better solutions for healing.

And to my beautiful children, Jordan and Jackson, for filling my heart with more love than I ever thought it was capable of holding. You provide my greatest lessons and inspiration. It is life with you that keeps me focused on what's most important. You two make up the biggest part of my *Why*.

REFERENCES

INTRODUCTION

1. Ruffing, V., Bingham, C., III. Rheumatoid arthritis signs and symptoms. Retrieved December, 2007, from http://www.hopkinsarthritis.org/arthritis-info/rheumatoid-arthritis/ra-symptoms/
2. Autoimmune statistics. Retrieved November 11, 2013, from http://www.aarda.org/autoimmune-information/autoimmune-statistics/
3. Chronic diseases and health promotion. (2014, May 09). Retrieved January 13, 2015, from http://www.cdc.gov/chronicdisease/overview/
4. Cleave, J. V., Gortmaker, S. L., & Perrin, J. M. (2010). Dynamics of obesity and chronic health conditions among children and youth. *The Journal of the American Medical Association, 303*(7), 623-630. Retrieved January 12, 2015.

CHAPTER 1

1. Rana, J. S., Nieuwdorp, M., Jukema, J. W., & Kastelein, J. J. (2007). Cardiovascular metabolic syndrome: an interplay

of, obesity, inflammation, diabetes and coronary heart disease. *Diabetes, Obesity and Metabolism, 9*(3), 218-232.

2. Coussens, L. M., & Werb, Z. (2002). Inflammation and cancer. *Nature, 420*(6917), 860-867.
3. Hyman, M. (2008). *The UltraMind solution: fix your broken brain by healing your body first: The simple way to defeat depression, overcome anxiety and sharpen your mind* (p. 175). New York: Scribner.
4. Noncommunicable diseases. (2015, January). Retrieved from http://www.who.int/mediacentre/factsheets/fs355/en/
5. Horton, R. (2015). Offline: Chronic diseases—the social justice issue of our time. *The Lancet, 386*(10011), 2378.
6. Challem, J. (2003). *The Inflammation Syndrome: The Complete Nutritional Program to Prevent and Reverse Heart Disease, Arthritis, Diabetes, Allergies and Asthma*. Hoboken, NJ: J. Wiley.
7. Fasano, A. (2011). Zonulin and its regulation of intestinal barrier function: the biological door to inflammation, autoimmunity, and cancer. *Physiological Reviews, 91*(1), 151-175. Retrieved June 5, 2015.
8. Matthews, J. (2014, July 14). *Bioindividual nutrition foundations*. Lecture presented at Bioindividual Nutrition Advanced Training for Practitioners.
9. Halis, G., & Arici, A. (2004). Endometriosis and inflammation in infertility. *Annals of the New York Academy of Sciences, 1034*(1), 300-315.

CHAPTER 2

1. Groff, J., Gropper, S. S., & Hunt, S. M. (1995). *Advanced nutrition and human metab*olism (2nd ed.). St. Paul, MN: West Publishing Company.
2. Human microbiome project. Retrieved 2014, from https://commonfund.nih.gov/hmp/index
3. Reid, A., & Greene, S. (2013). Human Microbiome (Rep.). American Academy of Microbiology.
4. Vighi, G., Marcucci, F., Sensi, L., Cara, G. D., & Frati, F. (2008). Allergy and the gastrointestinal system. *Clinical & Experimental Immunology, 153,* 3-6.
5. Gershon, M.D. (1995). The enteric system: A second brain. Hospital Practice, 34(7), 31-2.
6. Heijtz, R.D., Wang, S., Anuar, F., Qian, Y., Bjorkholm, B., Samuelson, A.,...Patterson, S. (2011). Normal gut microbiota modulates brain development and behavior. Proceedings of the National Academy of Sciences, 108(7), 3047-3052.
7. Mclean, M.H., Dieguez, D., Miller, L. & Young, H. A. (2014). Does the microbiota play a role in the pathogenesis of autoimmune diseases? Gut, 64(2), 332-41.
8. Visser, J., Rozing, J., Sapone, A., Lammers, K., & Fasano, A. (2009). Tight junctions, intestinal permeability, and autoimmunity. Annals of the New York Academy of Sciences, 1165(1), 195-205.
9. Fasano, A. (2011). Leaky gut and autoimmune diseases. Clinical Reviews in Allergy & Immunology Clinic Rev Allerg Immunol, 42(1), 71-78. Retrieved June 5, 2015.
10. A Protein in The Gut May Explain Why Some Can't Stomach Gluten. (2015, December 10). Retrieved 2016, from http://www.npr.org/sections/thesalt/2015/12/09/459061317/a-protein-in-the-gut-may-explain-why-some-cant-stomach-gluten

11. Snedeker, S. M., & Hay, A. G. (2011). Do interactions between gut ecology and environmental chemicals contribute to obesity and diabetes? Environmental Health Perspectives, 120(3), 332-339.

12. Fasano, A. (2011). Zonulin and its regulation of intestinal barrier function: the biological door to inflammation, autoimmunity, and cancer. Physiological Reviews, 91(1), 151-175. Retrieved June 5, 2015.

13. Katzka, D. (2007). The fecal microbiota of irritable bowel syndrome patients differs significantly from that of healthy subjects. *Gastroenterology, 133*(1), 24-33.

CHAPTER 3

1. Bayarsaihan, D. (2010). Epigenetic mechanisms in inflammation. *Journal of Dental Research,* 90(1), 9-17.

2. Genetics Home Reference. Retrieved December 2, 2015, from http://ghr.nlm.nih.gov/

3. Willett, W. C. (2002) Balancing life-style and genomics research for disease prevention. *Science,* 296(5568), 695-98.

4. Kaput, J., & Rodriguez, R. L. (2004). Nutritional genomics: The next frontier in the postgenomic era. *Physiol. Genomics Physiological Genomics, 16*(2), 166-177.

5. Kresser, C. (2015, February 24). Why your genes aren't your destiny. Retrieved February 25, 2015, from http://chriskresser.com/why-your-genes-arent-your-destiny/

6. Celeda, D., PhD. (2016). Clinical aspects of methylation. *The Integrative RDN, 18*(3), 68-71.

7. MTHFR. (2016). Retrieved April 19, 2016, from http://ghr.nlm.nih.gov/gene/MTHFR

8. MTHFR Gene Mutation. (2016). Retrieved April, 2016, from https://rarediseases.info.nih.gov/gard/10953/mthfr-gene-mutation/resources/9

9. Schmelzer, C., Lindner, I., Rimbach, G., Niklowitz, P., Menke, T., & Döring, F. (2008). Functions of coenzyme Q 10 in inflammation and gene expression. *BioFactors, 32*(1-4), 179-183.

CHAPTER 4

1. Pollan, M. (2006). The omnivore's dilemma: A natural history of four meals. New York: Penguin Press.

2. Pesticides. Retrieved October 10, 2015, from http://www.niehs.nih.gov/health/topics/agents/pesticides/

3. Environmental Impact. Retrieved April 10, 2014, from http://www.justlabelit.org/about-ge-foods-center/environmental-impact/

4. Seralini, G., Clair, E., Mesnage, R., Gress, S., Defarge, N., Malatesta, M., . . . Spiroux de Vandomois, J. (2014). Republished study: long-term toxicity of a Roundup herbicide and a Roundup-tolerant genetically modified maize. *Environmental Sciences Europe, 26*(14).

5. Mnif, W., Hassine, A. I., Bouaziz, A., Bartegi, A., Thomas, O., & Roig, B. (2011). Effect of endocrine disruptor pesticides: a review. *International Journal of Environmental Research and Public Health, 8*(12), 2265-2303.

6. Goldner, W. S., Sandler, D. P., Yu, F., Hoppin, J. A., Kamel, F., & Levan, T. D. (2010). Pesticide use and thyroid disease among women in the agricultural health study. *American Journal of Epidemiology, 171*(4), 455-464.

7. Orban, J. E., Stanley, J. S., Schwemberger, J. G., & Remmers, J. C. (1994). Dioxins and dibenzofurans in adipose tissue of the general US population and selected subpopulations. *American Journal of Public Health, 84*(3), 439-445.

8. Snedeker, S. M., & Hay, A. G. (2011). Do interactions between gut ecology and environmental chemicals contribute to obesity and diabetes? *Environmental Health Perspectives, 120*(3), 332-339.

9. Agricultural Marketing Service - Grass fed marketing claim standards. (2008, September 29). Retrieved January 21, 2015, from http://www.ams.usda.gov/AMSv1.0/ams.fetchTemplateData.do?template=TemplateN&rightNav1=GrassFedMarketingClaimStandards&topNav=&leftNav=GradingCertificationandVerfication&page=GrassFedMarketingClaims&resultType=

10. Labeling Around the World. Retrieved January 15, 2014, from http://www.justlabelit.org/right-to-know-center/labeling-around-the-world/

11. GMO Facts. Retrieved May 15, 2012, from http://www.nongmoproject.org/learn-more/

12. USDA ERS - Adoption of genetically engineered crops in the U.S.: recent trends in GE adoption. (2015, July 9). Retrieved October 19, 2015, from http://www.ers.usda.gov/data-products/adoption-of-genetically-engineered-crops-in-the-us/recent-trends-in-ge-adoption.aspx

13. Pollan, M. Modern Meat [Interview]. In *PBS*. Retrieved October 15, 2015.

14. Hyman, M., MD. (2009). The ecology of eating: the power of the fork. *Alternative Therapies in Health and Medicine,* 15(4), 14-15.

15. PCBs in Farmed Salmon. (2003, July 31). Retrieved October 15, 2015, from http://www.ewg.org/research/pcbs-farmed-salmon

16. PCB's in Farmed Salmon: Wild versus farmed. (2003, July 31). Retrieved October 10, 2015, from http://www.ewg.org/research/pcbs-farmed-salmon/wild-versus-farmed

17. PCBs cause cancer. Retrieved October 15, 2015, from http://www.ewg.org/research/pcbs-farmed-salmon/pcbs-cause-cancer

18. Ross, J. (2004). *The mood cure: The 4-step program to take charge of your emotions-today.* New York: Penguin.

19. Winter, R., M.S. (2009). *A Consumer's Dictionary of Food Additives*. New York: Three Rivers.

20. Generally Recognized as Safe – But is it? (2014, November 12). Retrieved February 05, 2015, from http://www.ewg.org/research/ewg-s-dirty-dozen-guide-food-additives/generally-recognized-as-safe-but-is-it

21. Kobylewski, S., & Jacobson, M. F., PhD. (2010). *Food dyes a rainbow of risks* (Rep.). Center for Science in the Public Interest.

22. Andrews, D. Synthetic ingredients in natural flavors and natural flavors in artificial flavors. Retrieved 2015, from http://www.ewg.org/foodscores/content/natural-vs-artificial-flavors

23. Food Additives Linked to Health Concerns. (2014, November 12). Retrieved 2014, from http://www.ewg.org/research/ewg-s-dirty-dozen-guide-food-additives/food-additives-linked-health-risks

24. International Agency for Research on Cancer. (2015). Q&A on the carcinogenicity of the consumption of red meat and processed meat. *International Agency for Research on Cancer.* World Health Organization. Retrieved, October 27, 2015.

25. Chambrun, G. P., Body-Malapel, M., Frey-Wagner, I., Djouina, M., Deknuydt, F., Atrott, K., . . . Vignal, C. (2013). Aluminum enhances inflammation and decreases mucosal healing in experimental colitis in mice. *Mucosal Immunology, 7*(3), 589-601.

26. Lerner, A. (2007). Aluminum Is a Potential Environmental Factor for Crohn's Disease Induction: Extended Hypothesis. *Annals of the New York Academy of Sciences, 1107*(1), 329-345.

27. Serrano, S. E., Braun, J., Trasande, L., Dills, R., & Sathyanarayana, S. (2014). Phthalates and diet: A review of the food monitoring and epidemiology data. *Environmental Health Environ Health, 13*(1), 43.

28. Salas, M., Nswosu, V.C. (2010). High fructose corn syrup: production, uses and public health concerns. *Biotechnology and Molecular Biology,* 5(5), 71-78.

29. Hyman, M., MD. (2011, May 13). 5 reasons high fructose corn syrup will kill you. Retrieved April, 2012, from http://drhyman.com/blog/2011/05/13/5-reasons-high-fructose-corn-syrup-will-kill-you/

30. Abou-Donia, M. B., El-Masry, E. M., Abdel-Rahman, A. A., Mclendon, R. E., & Schiffman, S. S. (2008). Splenda alters gut microflora and increases intestinal p-glycoprotein and cytochrome P-450 in Male Rats. *Journal of Toxicology and Environmental Health, Part A, 71*(21), 1415-1429.

31. Suez, J., Korem, T., Zeevi, D., Zilberman-Schapira, G., Thaiss, C. A., Maza, O., . . . Elinav, E. (2014). Artificial sweeteners induce glucose intolerance by altering the gut microbiota. *Nature,* 514(7521), 181-186.

CHAPTER 5

1. Davis, C., Saltos, E. (1999). Dietary recommendations and how they have changed over Time. *America's Eating Habits: Changes and Consequences.* Washington, DC: United States Department of Agriculture, 33-50.

2. Chang, C.Y., Ke, D.S., Chen, J.Y. (2009). Essential fatty acids and human brain. *Acta Neurol Taiwan,* 18(4), 230-41.

3. Enig, Mary G. (2000). *Know your fats: the complete primer for understanding the nutrition of fats, oils and cholesterol.* Silver Spring, MD: Bethesda.

4. Simopoulos, A.P. (2002). The importance of the ratio of omega-6/omega-3 essential fatty acids. *Biomedicine & Pharmacotherapy, 56(*8), 365-79.

5. Casal, S., Malheiro, R., Sendas, A., Oliveira, B. P., & Pereira, J. A. (2010). Olive oil stability under deep-frying conditions. *Food and Chemical Toxicology, 48*(10), 2972-2979.

6. Academy comments re The DGAC Scientific Report. (2015, May 8). Retrieved from http://www.eatrightpro.org/resource/news-center/on-the-pulse-of-public-policy/regulatory-comments/dgac-scientific-report

7. Healthy Eating Plate & Healthy Eating Pyramid. Retrieved 2014, from http://www.hsph.harvard.edu/nutritionsource/healthy-eating-plate/

8. Dinicolantonio, J. J., Lucan, S. C., & O'Keefe, J. H. (2016). The Evidence for saturated fat and for sugar related to coronary heart disease. Progress in Cardiovascular Diseases, 58(5), 464-472. doi:10.1016/j.pcad.2015.11.006

9. Draft Guidance for Industry and FDA Staff: Whole Grain Label Statements. (2006, February 17). Retrieved April, 2015, from http://www.fda.gov/Food/GuidanceRegulation/GuidanceDocumentsRegulatoryInformation/ucm059088.htm

10. Whole Grains. Retrieved April, 2015, from http://www.hsph.harvard.edu/nutritionsource/whole-grains

11. Gupta, S., MD (Writer). (2012, April 1). 60 Minutes [Television broadcast]. In *Is Sugar Toxic?* CBS.

12. Alexander, D. D., Weed, D. L., Cushing, C. A., & Lowe, K. A. (2011). Meta-analysis of prospective studies of red meat consumption and colorectal cancer. *European Journal of Cancer Prevention, 20*(4), 293-307.

13. Eckel, R. H., Jakicic, J. M., Ard, J. D., Jesus, J. M., Miller, N. H., Hubbard, V. S., . . . Yanovski, S. Z. (2013). 2013 AHA/ACC Guideline on lifestyle management to reduce cardiovascular risk. *Circulation, 129* (25 suppl 2)

14. Bonder, M. J., Tigchelaar, E. F., Cai, X., Trynka, G., Cenit, M. C., Hrdlickova, B., . . . Zhernakova, A. (2016). The influence of a short-term gluten-free diet on the human gut microbiome. *Genome Medicine, 8*(1), 45-55.

15. Micha, R., Wallace, S. K., & Mozaffarian, D. (2010). Red and

processed meat consumption and risk of incident coronary heart disease, stroke, and diabetes mellitus: a systematic review and meta-analysis. *Circulation, 121*(21), 2271-2283.

16. Lustwig, R., MD. (2014, May 2). Sugar: The Sweet Killer [Interview]. 2014 Food Revolution Summit.
17. Hybertson, B. M., Gao, B., Bose, S. K., & Mccord, J. M. (2011). Oxidative stress in health and disease: The therapeutic potential of Nrf2 activation. *Molecular Aspects of Medicine, 32*(4-6), 234-246.
18. Zhang, F. F., Morabia, A., Carroll, J., Gonzalez, K., Fulda, K., Kaur, M., . . . Cardarelli, R. (2011). Dietary patterns are associated with levels of global genomic DNA methylation in a cancer-free population. *Journal of Nutrition, 141*(6), 1165-1171.
19. Key, T. J., Thorogood, M., Appleby, P. N., & Burr, M. L. (1996). Dietary habits and mortality in 11,000 vegetarians and health conscious people: Results of a 17 year follow up. *British Medical Journal, 313*(7060), 775-779.
20. Hung, H. C., Joshipura, K. J., Jiang, R., Hu, F. B., Hunter, D., Smith-Warner, S., . . . Willett, W. (2004). Fruit and vegetable intake and major chronic disease. *J Natl Cancer Inst*, 96(21), 1577-1584.

CHAPTER 6

1. Guandalini, S., Newland, C. (2011). Differentiating food allergies from food intolerances. *Current Gastroenterology Reports,* 13(5), 426-34.
2. Ludvigsson, J. F., Montgomery, S. M., Ekbom, A., Brandt, L., & Granath, F. (2009). Small-intestinal histopathology and mortality risk in celiac disease. *The Journal of the American Medical Association, 302*(11), 1171-1178.
3. Farrell, R.J., Kelly, C.P. (2002). Celiac sprue. *New England Journal of Medicine* 346, 180-88.
4. Matthews, J. (2014, July 21). *Food Allergies and Sensitivi-*

ties and Gluten-Free/Casein-Free Diet. Lecture presented at Bioindividual Nutrition Advanced Training for Practitioners.

5. Pietzak, M. (2012). Celiac disease, wheat allergy, and gluten sensitivity: when gluten free is not a fad. *Journal of Parenteral and Enteral Nutrition, 36*(1 Suppl), 68S-75S.
6. Bizzaro, N., Tozzoli, R., Villalta, D., Fabris, M., & Tonutti, E. (2012). Cutting-edge issues in celiac disease and in gluten intolerance. *Clinical Reviews in Allergy & Immunology, 42*(3), 279-287.
7. Braly, J., Hoggan, R. (2002). *Dangerous grains: why gluten cereal grains may be hazardous to your health.* New York: Avery.
8. Samsel, A., Seneff, S. (2013). Glyphosate, pathways to modern diseases II: celiac sprue and gluten intolerance. *Interdisciplinary Toxicology,* 6*(*4), 159-84.
9. Kurokawa, Y., A. Maekawa, M. Takahashi, and Y. Hayashi. (1990). Toxicity and carcinogenicity of potassium bromate—a new renal carcinogen." *Environmental Health Perspectives,* 87, 309-35.
10. Food Additives Linked to Health Concerns. (2014, November 12). Retrieved February 10, 2014, from http://www.ewg.org/research/ewg-s-dirty-dozen-guide-food-additives/food-additives-linked-health-risks
11. Last eval.: Potassium Bromate (IARC Summary & Evaluation, Volume 73, 1999). (1999). Retrieved February 04, 2015, from http://www.inchem.org/documents/iarc/vol73/73-17.html
12. Potocki P, Hozyask K. (2002). Psychiatric symptoms and coeliac disease. *Psychiatr Pol*, 36(4), 567-78.
13. Galipeau, H. J., Mccarville, J. L., Huebener, S., Litwin, O., Meisel, M., Jabri, B., . . . Verdu, E. F. (2015). Intestinal microbiota modulates gluten-induced immunopathology in humanized mice. *The American Journal of Pathology,* 185(11), 2969-2982.

14. Pynnonen, P.A., Erkki, T., Isometsa, ET, Verkasalo, M.A., Kahkonen, S.A., Sipila, I.,... Aalberg, V.A. (2005) Gluten-free diet may alleviate depressive and behavioral symptoms in adolescents with coeliac disease. *BMC psychiatry*, 5-14.

15. Fukudome, S., Yoshikawa, M. (1992). Opioid peptides derived from wheat gluten: their isolation and characterization. *FEBS letters* 296(1), 107-111.

16. Kalaydijian A.E., Easton, W., Casella, N., Fasano, A. (2006). The gluten connection: the association between schizophrenia and celiac disease. *Acta Psychiatr Scan*, 113(2), 82-90.

17. Diagnosis & Testing - Food Allergy Research & Education. Retrieved May 18, 2014, from http://www.foodallergy.org/diagnosis-and-testing

18. Rubio-Tapia, A., Hill, I. D., Kelly, C. P., Calderwood, A. H., & Murray, J. A. (2013). ACG clinical guidelines: diagnosis and management of celiac disease. *The American Journal of Gastroenterology*, 108(5), 656-676.

19. Sapone, A., Bai, J. C., Ciacci, C., Dolinsek, J., Green, P. H., Hadjivassiliou, M., . . . Fasano, A. (2012). Spectrum of gluten-related disorders: Consensus on new nomenclature and classification. *BMC Medicine*, 10(1), 13.

20. Celiac Disease: On the Rise. (2010, July). Retrieved July 06, 2014, from http://www.mayo.edu/research/discoverys-edge/celiac-disease-rise

21. Screening - Celiac Disease Foundation. Retrieved June 15, 2014, from http://celiac.org/celiac-disease/diagnosing-celiac-disease/screening/

22. Teufel, A., Weinmann, A., Kahaly, G. J., Centner, C., Piendl, A., Wörns, M., . . . Kanzler, S. (2010). Concurrent autoimmune diseases in patients with autoimmune hepatitis. *Journal of Clinical Gastroenterology, 44*(3), 208-213.

23. Cusick, M. F., Libbey, J. E., & Fujinami, R. S. (2011). Molecular mimicry as a mechanism of autoimmune disease. *Clinical*

Reviews in Allergy & Immunology Clinic Rev Allerg Immunol, 42(1), 102-111.

24. Hartwig, A., Teschemacher, H., Lehmann, W., Gauly, M., Erhadt, G. (1997) Influence of genetic polymorphism in bovine milk on the occurence of bioactive peptides. *Milk Protein Polymorphism*, International Dairy Federation Special Publication, Brussels, Belgium, 9702, 459-460.
25. Jinsmaa, Y. & Yoshikawa, M. (1999) Enzymatic release of neocasomorphin and betacasomorphin from bovine beta-casein. *Peptides*, 20, 957-962.
26. Kamiński, S., Cieslińska, A. & Kostyra, E. (2007) Polymorphism of bovine beta-casein and its potential effect on human health. *The Journal of Applied Genetics*, 48(3):189-198.
27. Laugesen, M. & Elliot, R. (2003). Ischaemic heart disease, type 1 diabetes, and cow milk A1 -casein. *The New Zealand Medical Journal,* 116(1168), U295.
28. Monetini, L., Cavallo, M. G., Manfrini, S., Stefanini, L., Picarelli, A., Tola, M. D., . . . Pozzilli, P. (2002). Antibodies to bovine beta-casein in diabetes and other autoimmune diseases. *Hormone and Metabolic Research*, 34(8), 455-459.
29. Ganmaa, D., Xiaohui, C., Feskanich, D, Hankinson, S. & Willett, W. (2011). "Milk, dairy intake and risk of endometrial cancer: a 26-year follow-up. *International Journal of Cancer Int. J. Cancer*, 11, 2664-671.
30. Weil, A., MD. Does milk cause cancer. Retrieved October 01, 2015, from http://www.drweil.com/drw/u/QAA400175/Does-Milk-Cause-Cancer.html
31. Reichelt, K., Jensen, D. (2004). IgA antibodies against gliadin and gluten in multiple sclerosis. *Acta neurologica scandinavica,* 110(4), 239-241.
32. Wasilewska, J., Sienkiewicz-Szłapka, E., Kuźbida, E., Jarmołowska, B., Kaczmarski, M., & Kostyra, E. (2011). The ex-

ogenous opioid peptides and DPPIV serum activity in infants with apnoea expressed as apparent life threatening events (ALTE). *Neuropeptides, 45*(3), 189-195.

33. Hallert, C., Åström, J., & Sedvall, G. (1982). Psychic disturbances in adult coeliac disease. *Scand J Gastroenterol Scandinavian Journal of Gastroenterology, 17*(1), 25-28.

34. Zueroro-Casano, G., Moreno-Rojas, R., & Amaro-Lopez, M. (1994). Effect of processing on contents and relationships of mineral elements of milk. *Food Chemistry, 51*(1), 75-78.

35. Dhiman, T., Anand, G., Satter, L., & Pariza, M. (1999). Conjugated linoleic acid content of milk from cows fed different diets. *Journal of Dairy Science, 82*(10), 2146-2156.

36. Kresser, C. (2012, May 18). Raw milk reality: benefits of raw milk. Retrieved September 15, 2015, from http://chriskresser.com/raw-milk-reality-benefits-of-raw-milk/

37. Forristal, L. J. (2004, May 23). Ultra-pasteurized milk - Weston A Price. Retrieved September 15, 2015, from http://www.westonaprice.org/health-topics/ultra-pasteurized-milk/

38. Michaelsson, K., Wolk, A., Langenskiold, S., Basu, S., Lemming, E. W., Melhus, H., & Byberg, L. (2014). Milk intake and risk of mortality and fractures in women and men: Cohort studies. *British Medical Journal*, 349 (Oct27 1).

39. Radford, L. T., Bolland, M. J., Mason, B., Horne, A., Gamble, G. D., Grey, A., & Reid, I. R. (2013). The Auckland calcium study: 5-year post-trial follow-up. *Osteoporosis International, 25*(1), 297-304.

40. Matthews, J. (2014, July 21). *Dysbiosis and Diets for GI Support.* Lecture presented at Bioindividual Nutrition Advanced Training for Practitioners.

CHAPTER 7

1. Qi, Z., Hoffman, G., Kurtycz, D., & Yu, J. (2003). Prevalence of the C677T substitution of the methylenetetrahydrofolate reductase (MTHFR) gene in Wisconsin. *Genetics in Medicine Genet Med, 5*(6), 458-459.

2. Celeda, D., PhD. (2016). Clinical aspects of methylation. *The Integrative RDN, 18*(3), 68-71.

3. Trade Secrets: A Moyers Report [Interview by B. Moyer & S. Jones, Transcript]. PBS.

4. Harley, K. G., Kogut, K., Madrigal, D. S., Cardenas, M., Vera, I. A., Meza-Alfaro, G., . . Parra, K. L. (2016). Reducing phthalate, paraben, and phenol exposure from personal care products in adolescent girls: findings from the HERMOSA intervention study. *Environmental Health Perspectives.* doi:10.1289/ehp.1510514

5. Fragrance in Cosmetics. (2015, December 29). Retrieved April, 2015, from http://www.fda.gov/cosmetics/productsingredients/ingredients/ucm388821.htm#phthalates

6. Parabens. Retrieved April 27, 2015, from http://www.ewg.org/sites/humantoxome/chemicals/chemical_classes.php?-class=Parabens

7. Kwak, E. S., Just, A., Whyatt, R., & Miller, R. L. (2009). Phthalates, pesticides, and bisphenol-a exposure and the development of nonoccupational asthma and allergies: how valid are the links? *The Open Allergy Journal, 2*(1), 45-50.

8. Serrano, S. E., Braun, J., Trasande, L., Dills, R., & Sathyanarayana, S. (2014). Phthalates and diet: A review of the food monitoring and epidemiology data. *Environmental Health Environ Health, 13*(1), 43.

9. Zota, A. R., Phillips, C. A., & Mitro, S. D. (2016). Recent fast food consumption and bisphenol A and phthalates exposures

among the U.S. population in NHANES, 2003–2010. *EHP Environmental Health Perspectives*. doi: 10.1289/ehp.1510803

10. Stejskal, V., Ockert, K., Bjorklund, G. (2013). Metal-induced inflammation triggers fibromyalgia in metal-allergic patients. *Neuro Endocrinol Lett,* 34(6), 559-65.
11. Aminzadeh, K.K., Etminan, M. (2007) Dental Amalgam and Multiple Sclerosis: A Systematic Review and Meta-Analysis. *Journal of Public Health Dentistry,* 67 (1), 64-66.
12. Azevedo, B. F., Furieri, L. B., Peçanha, F. M., Wiggers, G. A., Vassallo, P. F., Simões, M. R., . . . Vassallo, D. V. (2012). Toxic effects of mercury on the cardiovascular and central nervous systems. *Journal of Biomedicine and Biotechnology, 2012*, 1-11.
13. Dórea, J., Marques, R., & Brandão, K. (2009). Neonate exposure to thimerosal mercury from Hepatitis B vaccines. *Amer J Perinatol American Journal of Perinatology, 26*(07), 523-527.
14. Mannello, F., Tonti, G. A., Medda, V., Simone, P., & Darbre, P. D. (2011). Analysis of aluminum content and iron homeostasis in nipple aspirate fluids from healthy women and breast cancer-affected patients. *Journal of Applied Toxicology, 31*(3), 262-269.
15. Sears, M. E., Kerr, K. J., & Bray, R. I. (2012). Arsenic, cadmium, lead, and mercury in sweat: a systematic eview. *Journal of Environmental and Public Health*, 2012, 1-10.
16. Hyman, M., MD. (2010, May 19). How to Rid Your Body of Heavy Metals: A 3-Step Detoxification Plan - Dr. Mark Hyman. Retrieved April, 2014, from http://drhyman.com/blog/2010/05/19/how-to-rid-your-body-of-mercury-and-other-heavy-metals-a-3-step-plan-to-recover-your-health/
17. Kresser, C. (2010, July 29). The Thyroid-Gut Connection. Retrieved April, 2015, from http://chriskresser.com/the-thyroid-gut-connection/
18. *Dirty Dozen List of Endocrine Disruptors: 12 Hormone-Altering Chemicals and How to Avoid Them* (Publication). (2013). Retrieved

April 27, 2014, from EWG and Keep A Breast website: http://www.ewg.org/research/dirty-dozen-list-endocrine-disruptors

19. Lamas, G. A., Goertz, C., Boineau, R., Mark, D. B., Rozema, T., Nahin, R. L., . . . Investigators, F. T. (2013). Effect of disodium EDTA chelation regimen on cardiovascular events in patients with previous myocardial infarction. *Journal of the American Medical Association,* 309(12), 1241-1250.

20. NTP Finalizes Report on Bisphenol A. (2008, September 3). Retrieved 2015, from http://www.niehs.nih.gov/news/newsroom/releases/2008/september03/

21. Healthy Home Tips: Tip 3 - Pick Plastics Carefully. Retrieved 2015, from http://www.ewg.org/research/healthy-home-tips/tip-3-pick-plastics-carefully

22. Okada, H., Kuhn, C., Feillet, H., & Bach, J. (2010). The 'hygiene hypothesis' for autoimmune and allergic diseases: An update. *Clinical & Experimental Immunology, 160*(1), 1-9.

23. Nailed: Nail polish chemical doubles as furniture fire retardant. (2015, October 19). Retrieved April, 2015, from http://www.ewg.org/research/nailed/nail-polish-chemical-doubles-furniture-fire-retardant

24. Silverman, M.N. & Sternberg, E.M. (2012). Glucocorticoid regulation of inflammation and its functional correlates: from HPA axis to glucocorticoid receptor dysfunction." *Annals of the New York Academy of Sciences,* 1261(1), 55-63.

25. Kresser, C. (2016, March 16). *Overcoming adrenal fatigue.* Lecture.

26. Powell, N. D., Sloan, E. K., Bailey, M. T., Arevalo, J. M., Miller, G. E., Chen, E., . . . Cole, S. W. (2013). Social stress up-regulates inflammatory gene expression in the leukocyte transcriptome via -adrenergic induction of myelopoiesis. *Proceedings of the National Academy of Sciences, 110*(41), 16574-16579.

27. Vanuytsel, T., Wanrooy, S. V., Vanheel, H., Vanormelingen, C.,

Verschueren, S., Houben, E., . . . Tack, J. (2013). Psychological stress and corticotropin-releasing hormone increase intestinal permeability in humans by a mast cell-dependent mechanism. *Gut, 63*(8), 1293-1299.

28. Mullington, J. M., Simpson, N. S., Meier-Ewert, H. K., & Haack, M. (2010). Sleep loss and inflammation. *Best Practice & Research Clinical Endocrinology & Metabolism, 24*(5), 775-784.

29. Irwin, M. R., Wang, M., Ribeiro, D., Cho, H. J., Olmstead, R., Breen, E. C., . . . Cole, S. (2008). Sleep loss activates cellular inflammatory signaling. *Biological Psychiatry, 64*(6), 538-540.

30. Chang, A., Santhi, N., Hilaire, M. S., Gronfier, C., Bradstreet, D. S., Duffy, J. F., . . . Czeisler, C. A. (2012). Human responses to bright light of different durations. *The Journal of Physiology, 590*(13), 3103-3112.

31. Epstein, Z. (2014, May 29). Horrifying chart reveals how much time we spend staring at screens each day. Retrieved April 28, 2015, from http://bgr.com/2014/05/29/smartphone-computer-usage-study-chart/

CHAPTER 8

1. Neu, J., & Rushing, J. (2011). Cesarean versus vaginal delivery: long-term infant outcomes and the hygiene hypothesis. *Clinics in Perinatology, 38*(2), 321-331.

2. Hamilton, B. E., Martin, J. A., Osterman, M. J., Curtin, S. C., & Matthews, T. (2015). Births: final data for 2014. *National Vital Statistics Reports, 64*(12), 1-63.

3. Blaser, M. J., & Falkow, S. (2009). What are the consequences of the disappearing human microbiota? *Nature Reviews Microbiology, 7*(12), 887-894.

4. Newburg, D.S., Walker, W.A,.(2007). Protection of the neo-

nate by the innate immune system of developing gut and of human milk. *Pediatric Research*, 6, 2-8.

5. Jackson, M., Nazar, A.M. (2006). Breastfeeding, the immune response and long-term health. The *Journal of the American Osteopathic Association,* 106, 203-207.

6. Blaser, M. (2011). Antibiotic overuse: stop the killing of beneficial bacteria. *Nature, 476*(7361), 393-394. Retrieved May 17, 2015.

7. Chutkan, Robynne, MD. Proc. of Women's Health and the Environment Myth Busting Media Briefing, Washington, D.C. Environmental Working Group, 16 Sept. 2015. Web.

8. Sigthorsson, G., Tibble, J., Hayllar, J., Menzies, I., Macpherson, A., Moots, R., . . . Bjarnason, I. (1998, October). Intestinal permeability and inflammation in patients on NSAIDs. Retrieved May 17, 2015, from http://www.ncbi.nlm.nih.gov/pmc/articles/PMC1727292/

9. Duke, J.A. (2007). The Garden Pharmacy: Turmeric, the queen of COX-2-inhibitors. *Alternative and Complementary Therapies,* 13(5), 229-34.

10. Bost, J., Maroon, A., & Maroon, J. (2010). Natural anti-inflammatory agents for pain relief. *Surgical Neurology International Surg Neurol Int, 1*(1), 80.

11. Ibuprofen: MedlinePlus Drug Information. Retrieved May 17, 2015, from http://www.nlm.nih.gov/medlineplus/druginfo/meds/a682159.html

12. Fasano, A. (2011). Zonulin and its regulation of intestinal barrier function: the biological door to inflammation, autoimmunity, and cancer. *Physiological Reviews, 91*(1), 151-175. Retrieved June 5, 2015.

13. Seto, C. T., Jeraldo, P., Orenstein, R., Chia, N., & Dibaise, J. K. (2014). Prolonged use of a proton pump inhibitor reduces microbial diversity: Implications for Clostridium difficile

susceptibility. *Microbiome, 2*(1), 42.

14. Lu, B., Solomon, D. H., Costenbader, K. H., Keenan, B. T., Chibnik, L. B., & Karlson, E. W. (2010). Alcohol consumption and markers of inflammation in women with preclinical rheumatoid arthritis. *Arthritis & Rheumatism, 62*(12), 3554-3559.

15. Wang, H. J. (2010). Alcohol, inflammation, and gut-liver-brain interactions in tissue damage and disease development. *World Journal of Gastroenterology WJG, 16*(11), 1304-1313.

16. Weiss, M., M.D. (2011, November 9). Alcohol and Cancer: You Can't Drink to Your Health. Retrieved April, 2015, from http://community.breastcancer.org/livegreen/alcohol-and-cancer-you-cant-drink-to-your-health/

17. Lee, J., Taneja, V., & Vassallo, R. (2011). Cigarette smoking and inflammation: cellular and molecular mechanisms. *Journal of Dental Research, 91*(2), 142-149.

18. Health Effects of Cigarette Smoking. (2015, October 01). Retrieved April, 2016, from http://www.cdc.gov/tobacco/data_statistics/fact_sheets/health_effects/effects_cig_smoking/#children

19. Pelton, R., LaValle, J. B., & Hawkins, E. B. (2001). *Drug-induced nutrient depletion handbook.* Hudson, OH: Lexi-Comp.

CHAPTER 9

1. Villa, R., & Thousand, J. (1999). A framework for thinking about systems change. In T. Knoster (Author), *Restructuring for Caring and Effective Education: Piecing the Puzzle Together* (p. 97). Paul H. Brookes Publishing.

2. Bergland, C. (2011, December 26). The Neuroscience of Perseverance. Retrieved October, 2015, from https://www.psychologytoday.comhttps://www.psychologytoday.com/blog/the-athletes-way/201112/the-neuroscience-perseverance/

blog/the-athletes-way/201112/the-neuroscience-perseverance

CHAPTER 10

1. Academy Comments re The DGAC Scientific Report. (2015, May 8). Retrieved from http://www.eatrightpro.org/resource/news-center/on-the-pulse-of-public-policy/regulatory-comments/dgac-scientific-report
2. EWG's updated water filter buying guide. (2013, February 27). Retrieved from http://www.ewg.org/research/ewgs-water-filter-buying-guide
3. Barański, M., Średnicka-Tober, D., Volakakis, N., Seal, C., Sanderson, R., Stewart, G. B., . . . Leifert, C. (2014). Higher antioxidant and lower cadmium concentrations and lower incidence of pesticide residues in organically grown crops: A systematic literature review and meta-analyses. *British Journal of Nutrition, 112*(05), 794-811.
4. Matthews, J. (2014, July 21). *Dysbiosis and Diets for GI Support.* Lecture presented at Bioindividual Nutrition Advanced Training for Practitioners.
5. Goel, N., Kim, H., & Lao, R. P. (2005). An olfactory stimulus modifies nighttime sleep in young men and women. *Chronobiology International*, 22(5), 889-904.
6. Lee, I.S., Lee, G.J. (2006). Effects of lavender aromatherapy on insomnia and depression in women college students. Taehan Kanho Hakhoe Chi, 36(1), 136-43.
7. Jacobs, D. R., Gross, M. D., & Tapsell, L. C. (2009). Food synergy: An operational concept for understanding nutrition. *American Journal of Clinical Nutrition*, 89(5).
8. Kliger, B., Cohrssen, A. (2008). Probiotics" *American Family*

Physician, 78(9), 1073-8.

9. Fallon, S., & Enig, M. G., Ph.D. (2015, November 23). Cod Liver Oil Basics and Recommendations. Retrieved 2014, from http://www.westonaprice.org/health-topics/cod-liver-oil-basics-and-recommendations/
10. Tolle, E. (1999). The power of now: A guide to spiritual enlightenment (pp. 84-85). Novato, CA: New World Library.

EPILOGUE

1. Westfall, J. M., Mold, J., & Fagnan, L. (2007). Practice-based research—"blue highways" on the NIH Roadmap. *Journal of the American Medical Association*, 297(4), 403.
2. Murray, C. J., Phil, D., & Frenk, J. (2010, January 14). Ranking 37th - Measuring the Performance of the U.S. Health Care System — NEJM. Retrieved June 10, 2014, from http://www.nejm.org/doi/full/10.1056/NEJMp0910064
3. Italy, United Nations. (2013). *The state of food and agriculture 2013 food systems for better nutrition*. Rome: FAO
4. Wahls, T., M.D. (2014, September 15). "*Evolutionary Nutrition: Recovering from MS and Autoimmune Disease*. Lecture presented at The Evolution of Medicine Summit.

INDEX

A

B

C

D

E

F

G

H

I

J

K

L

M

N

O

P

Q

R

S

T

U

V

W

Z

Made in the USA
San Bernardino, CA
22 July 2018